What People Are Saying About

Natural Happiness

Natural Happiness is inspiring and practical. Based on decades of hands-on experience, Alan Heeks entwines gardening strategies with mindful exercises that are proven to improve your wellbeing. His approach also has a poetic and ecologically sensitive side as he draws parallels between our personal challenges and the fragile state of Gaia our planet. If you are looking for a helpful, grounded and realistic approach; if you love nature and gardening; if you want to improve your wellbeing — then this short and friendly book is for you.

Dr William Bloom, international author and educator

If you wanted to improve your life by growing just one thing, what would you choose? 'Yourself' is Alan's answer and I agree. He's mapped out so beautifully how we can do this, growing not only our wellbeing and resilience, but also our rootedness in the world. As someone who's inspired by projects Alan has developed, I'm so pleased he's sharing his practical vision and approach in this book.

Dr Chris Johnstone, co-author of *Active Hope*, leading expert in resilience and wellbeing

Alan Heeks' wise book offers subtle but powerful ways to restore happiness in our lives. We can cultivate wellbeing like gardeners cultivate their gardens, noticing the essentials — soil, sun, air, compost and water — and making small adjustments to increase a vibrancy. Our happiness can grow as we tend, rather than fix, what ails us.

Vicki Robin, leading US author and social innovator

I love how Alan takes the positives of gardening and translates them to everyday life, with phrases such as compost your troubles and cultivate community. He shows how to translate the practicalities of life-affirming garden methods into our own lives, which sets up a loop of positive feedback between us and plants. Grow a green finger, healthy plants, great soil and feel vibrant while doing it.

Charles Dowding, leading UK organic gardener and author

Alan's wise and joyous celebratory book shows how our primordial relationship with our planetary home Gaia is not only fundamental to our healing within ourselves and each other, but vital to our potential to survive and thrive — and to consciously evolve — as a planetary and universal species.

Dr Jude Currivan, cosmologist, planetary healer, author, co-founder of WholeWorld-View

New evidence from the Amazon to Australia tells us that we humans were improving the biodiversity and food productivity of wildernesses for thousands of years before the start of sedentary agriculture. In other words, we are a gardening species. That might be why we can feel so at home and at peace when gardening today. And it is why we can approach gardening with a renewed reverence and confidence. Alan Heeks taps into this truth as he advises on how gardening yourself can be as meaningful, healing and celebratory as possible. Your harvests will be even more enjoyable after reading this book.

Professor Jem Bendell, initiator of the Deep Adaptation Forum

I have worked with Alan for over ten years as a valued fellow of the Schumacher Institute. His passion to help people and address the big questions of the future — the climate crisis, biodiversity loss, and community resilience — is an inspiration. This book draws together much of his thinking on ways that nature and gardening can provide powerful answers, both literal and metaphorical, to generate happiness.
Ian Roderick, Director, The Schumacher Institute

Natural Happiness

Use Organic Gardening Skills
to Cultivate Yourself

Natural Happiness

Use Organic Gardening Skills
to Cultivate Yourself

Alan Heeks

BOOKS

Winchester, UK
Washington, USA

JOHN HUNT PUBLISHING

First published by O-Books, 2024
O-Books is an imprint of John Hunt Publishing Ltd., 3 East St., Alresford,
Hampshire SO24 9EE, UK
office@jhpbooks.com
www.johnhuntpublishing.com
www.o-books.com

For distributor details and how to order please visit the 'Ordering' section on our website.

Text copyright: Alan Heeks 2023

ISBN: 978 1 80341 496 6
978 1 80341 497 3 (ebook)
Library of Congress Control Number: 2023931819

A CIP catalogue record for this book is available from the British Library.

Design: Lapiz Digital Services

UK: Printed and bound by CPI Group (UK) Ltd, Croydon, CR0 4YY
Printed in North America by CPI GPS partners

The author of this book does not dispense medical advice or
prescribe the use of any technique as a form of treatment for
physical, emotional, or medical problems without the advice of a
physician, either directly or indirectly. The intent of the author
is only to offer information of a general nature to help you in
your quest for emotional and spiritual well-being. In the event
you use any of the information in this book for yourself, which is
your constitutional right, the author and the publisher assume no
responsibility for your actions.

We operate a distinctive and ethical publishing philosophy in
all areas of our business, from our global network of authors to
production and worldwide distribution.

Contents

Chapter 1 Nourish Your Roots　　　　　　　　　1
How this book can help you. Try the tree talk — are your roots, trunk and branches in balance? How to cultivate your ground condition: the underlying resources that feed your roots and wellbeing. The stories behind the book.

Chapter 2 Use Natural Energy Sources　　　　16
Learn to harness clean energy sources like appreciation, instead of polluting and depleting energy from stress, caffeine, etc. The four elements of natural energy, and tips for personal regeneration. Apply gardening methods like pruning, mulching, and seasonal cycles to your life and work.

Chapter 3 Compost Your Troubles　　　　　　40
In natural systems, waste becomes a major source of energy for growth. See how to transform negative feelings and problem situations by composting them. Constructive ways to process conflicts, using natural communication. Changing the Story: ways to uproot negative patterns.

Chapter 4 Shaping Uncertainty: The Co-creative Way　　60
Bewildering situations need new skills like co-creativity, tracker vision, Fox Walk, deep listening and the Diamond Process. Learn how to befriend your problems, get creative help from Nature, and manifest your hopes.

Chapter 5 Cultivating Community　　　　　　80
See how natural systems thrive on mutual support, and use diversity and wild margins. Understanding different

kinds of community, and how to work with them, including neighbourhood groups. Projects to learn from, and a community-building toolkit.

Chapter 6 Growing through Climate Change   101
How to face rising turbulence. Ways we can learn from Nature and support her. Choosing natural regeneration over techno-fixes. Useful frameworks such as Deep Ecology and Deep Adaptation. Perspectives, big questions and how to find your focus.

Chapter 7 Natural Inspiration   125
How Nature can help you find faith and a bigger perspective. Drawing guidance and support from your garden: connection, attunement. Soul connection, self-care, applied inspiration.

Appendix: Resource Toolkit   141
Processes and insights to help you go deeper, including Personal Energy Audit, Circle of Voices, and Community Insights.

Acknowledgements   152
About Alan Heeks   153
Keep Growing with Alan   154
Other Books by Alan Heeks   155

This book is dedicated to Mother Earth, Gaia, who nourishes our bodies and souls, with a hope that humanity realises its oneness with all life, and that we grow through this together.

Chapter 1

Nourish Your Roots

This book shows you how we can grow our own happiness, even in these uncertain times: by cultivating our human nature as a gardener tends their garden. Organic gardens and farms use regenerative methods that have clear parallels for people: such as composting, mulching, and observation skills. Life in the 2020s can be pretty overwhelming, but *Natural Happiness* offers you simple, practical ways to lift your spirits in this stormy season.

We're living in such turmoil that it may be hard to believe there are upsides to the challenges, but I invite you to try. This could be a chance to live more simply, more locally, to grow mutual support in your neighbourhood. You could treat the stress as an invitation to learn new skills, such as Deep Adaptation and organic resilience. Parallels with gardening give us easy ways to explore all this.

For example, a tree under stress will deepen its roots, so it reaches out further for water and nutrients, and to access the network of mutual support with fungal mycelium and other trees. This offers a useful parallel for us humans, and you can guide and motivate your resilience by imagining you have roots, just like a tree. Try it, later in this chapter!

Since 2020, we've had a series of emergencies piled on each other: Covid, Ukraine, energy shortages and more. Where's it heading? It's safe to say that we have to live with rising uncertainties on many fronts. We've hit the limits of growth on this planet: the future will bring shortages of energy, food, water, and so on. But we have choices: we can choose to adapt and co-operate, or we can fight each other for the last loaf. All ecosystems thrive on symbiosis, meaning every element gives

1

what it can, so the collective is stronger than the parts. This points to the deeper, organic communities we humans need to grow.

People sometimes compare themselves to a complex mechanism, like a car or computer, but that's too simplistic. We are living organisms, like a garden. I've found that *cultivated natural ecosystems*, such as a garden or organic farm, are the best guide to growing our own happiness: showing us how to steer an organism to a positive outcome using natural growth methods. I call this approach the Gardener's Way: it's easy to use, whether you're a gardener or not. The parallels are simple, and all explained in the book.

In The Gardener's Way, see yourself as both the garden and the gardener. You are a natural organism, like the garden: and you're also the gardener, who brings love and brains to cultivate the earth. It's clear that you can't understand a garden from a purely physical point of view. Feelings, intuition, inspiration are involved. Natural Happiness can guide you to bring these subtler qualities into your work, your home life, and into groups and community projects.

The roots of this book are back in the 1990s, when I moved from a successful career in business management to starting an organic farm from scratch: it was a huge shock. I was trained to take control and make things happen. Soon I learned that in organic farms and gardens, you control nothing: you have to co-create *with* the realities of the situation. These are the kind of skills I'll share in this book: how to dance with uncertainty, and steer a system you don't control towards the outcomes you'd like.

It's very easy to feel confused and helpless these days, as the crises pile up, and we're deluged with fake news and social media. *Natural Happiness* enables you to deepen your own roots, your own reality, drawing on the practical, delightful world of gardening.

How This Book Can Help You

This is a practical guide to growing your own happiness. There are no instant fixes, but this book offers a grounded, practical approach which you can easily learn. It will help you to understand how human nature works and how to cultivate it, like a gardener, using natural principles. For example:

- Deepening your roots and resilience
- Finding new sources of natural energy
- Composting difficulties, to provide fresh insights and momentum
- Strengthening your co-creative skills, so you handle problems more positively
- Growing support and resilience in groups such as your local community
- Evolving positive approaches to big issues, especially climate change

One of the best ways to improve your happiness is to strengthen your resilience: the ability to handle challenges and stress in a positive way, so that you bounce back and grow through them. It's very different from coping or getting by, which usually leave us anxious and subdued. The Gardener's Way offers you a set of resilient life skills which should really help your general mood and wellbeing.

I realised many years ago that I was less happy than I could be, and all the methods in this book were learned in my personal journey. I tend to worry and get unsettled by challenges in my own life and the wider world. My antidote came by noticing how gardeners and organic farmers handle uncertainties: they nourish deep resilience in themselves and in their land. This can be the roots your happiness grows from.

Chapters 1–3 will show you ways to cultivate the roots of your resilience, harnessing natural energy, and composting your troubles. From Chapter 4 onwards, we'll explore how to cultivate your growth, and your relation to the wider world, starting with co-creative skills in Chapter 4.

Life is getting more complex and demanding for most of us, so we're going to need better ways to co-operate in groups and communities, and more ability to handle friction and conflict with others. Chapter 5 can help you with new skills in those areas, using parallels from organic gardening, like valuing the wild margins.

Many people's happiness is affected by worries about the state of the world, and issues like climate change, which can leave us feeling overwhelmed and despairing. In Chapter 6 you'll find ways to handle these feelings differently, grow through them, and explore how you can make a positive contribution. Finally, Chapter 7 explores how to find a sense of purpose and perspective through inspiration from Nature.

Nourish Your Roots: Try the Tree Talk

Each chapter of this book explores one of the Seven Seeds of Natural Happiness. This short exercise introduces the first one: it shows you the benefits of balancing your system and deepening your roots. A tree offers a beautifully simple model of harmony between three main elements, as shown below.

A gardener knows that these three parts of the system must be balanced. If the branches are too extensive, the tree is physically unstable and risks depletion, so the branches would need pruning. If the root system isn't large enough to support the outputs you want, adding mulch and nutrients can help to reinforce it.

The tree talk is simply imagining yourself like a tree, and asking if these three elements of your system are in balance. Be aware that the resources you take in and use are not only physical: you're also drawing on emotional energy, such as appreciation, and inspirational energy, such as vision and hope.

Ideally, do this process outdoors, sitting or standing at the base of a tree. If that's hard, at least picture a tree you like. Slowly imagine these three elements of your system in turn, from the roots up, as if you were a tree.

Your roots: do you have a good support network (inner resources, outer contacts) that give you stability in challenges? Does your 'root network' extend enough to draw in energy and nourishment to sustain your outputs?

Your trunk: the trunk represents the ways you use energy to create what you want and adapt to change. Are your ways effective, stable and flexible?

Your branches/ fruits: do you feel your branches are over-extended in relation to your roots and trunk, or could they support you producing more outputs, more fruit?

Branches – fruits: the network of branches carry leaves which capture sunlight and which breathe, transforming carbon dioxide into oxygen. And this is where fruits, blossom and other outputs are produced.

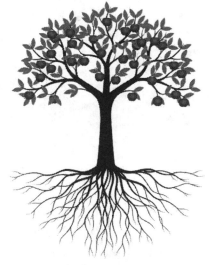

Trunk: the trunk has to combine stability and flexibility. It raises the crown, the higher branches, up to catch the light, but it must be able to bend with the wind. The trunk is the core of the tree, linking roots and branches.

Roots: the tree's roots give it physical stability against high winds, by anchoring it broadly in the earth. And they give access to resources: the network of roots takes in moisture and nutrients from the soil.

Use this dialogue to see where your system may need balancing: for example, by nourishing your roots or pruning your branches. There are tips on doing this below, and in Chapter 2.

I've guided hundreds of people through the tree talk in my workshops, from ultra-stressed hospital doctors to bewildered teenagers. It may sound odd, but it works. If you can get up close with a physical tree (or even just visualise a tree), relax, and start to feel that you are a natural organism just like the tree, insights will come. This process is a useful pointer for the rest of the book: the more you can imagine yourself as a garden, and its gardener, the more you'll find intuitions arising organically.

Mini Case Study: Lizzie

Lizzie came on one of my workshops, complaining of burnout. She was trying to juggle starting a design business with a new relationship, and parenting a young son by her previous partner. In the tree test, she saw herself as a big tree buffeted by gales, at risk of blowing right over or losing a large branch. She saw her roots as too small for this large, over-extended tree under stress. Deepening her roots would help: this could mean asking for more help from her parents and friends, and somehow making time to care for herself. Lizzie saw that she was giving out on all fronts, and decided she had to put the new relationship on hold: 'If he really cares, he'll wait. That image of a big branch torn off has to be taken seriously.'

Improving Your Ground Condition

Ground condition is a vital issue for gardeners and organic farmers. In a cultivated natural system, the key measure of success is not outputs and results, it's the state of the soil. The vitality and resilience of ground condition provides the resources to handle unexpected problems and keep growing in future. It's a valuable approach for human nature too.

If this idea feels odd, let's explore a different angle on it. Mainstream farming could mostly be called industrial or forced farming: crop growth comes from artificial fertilisers, *not* from the underlying vitality of the soil. Over time, these fertilisers, and related pesticides, pollute the earth and lower its vitality and its resilience to such problems as droughts or diseases. This means the gardener or farmer becomes ever more dependent on artificial stimulants and suppressants. Domestic vegetable gardens may have similar issues, but the difference between mainstream and organic is not so marked.

Can you see the parallel in human nature? Many people push themselves along with artificial, polluting habits like stress, comfort food, caffeine, alcohol and lots more. This depletes their ground condition, and lowers their resilience to new challenges. The alternative is to nourish your ground condition, and value both roots and fruits. As Lady Eve Balfour, an organic farming pioneer, put it: 'Feed the soil, and the soil will feed the plant.'

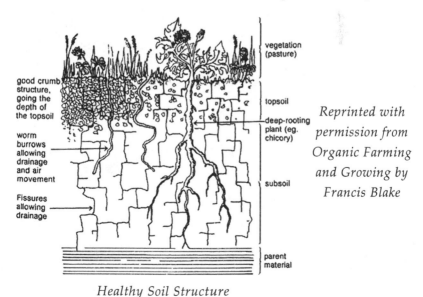

Reprinted with permission from Organic Farming and Growing by *Francis Blake*

Healthy Soil Structure

Have a look at this diagram of healthy soil. One of the important features of fertile ground condition is structure. Good structure is permeable, so that air, heat and water can get into the soil, and excess water can drain through it. It has enough openness that roots can penetrate down, and enough strength to support root structures firmly.

The most common structural problem with soil is *compaction*. This means that the soil is too dense: air, water and warmth can't circulate, and so fertility drops. I meet a lot of people I'd call compacted: you might call them uptight or tense. One benefit of the analogy is that if you really imagine you're compacted earth, this can lead you to remedies. You may feel how you need to relax, open up to let resources in and feed your roots.

Self-help Quickie: Handling Compaction

This self-guided process should only take about 10 minutes. Read these instructions a couple of times, then work from memory as much as possible.

Find a quiet place where you can sit upright but relaxed. Get yourself comfortable, and close your eyes.

Take some long, slow breaths. On the outbreath, push out any tension you're feeling, park any worrying thoughts.

Now imagine your body like a garden with compacted soil. Really feel the tensions in your body as if this is hard, dense earth. And just as a gardener listens to the land, listen to what your body needs. How can you help it?

Take some really long, slow breaths, as deep as you can: imagine you're relaxing the tension, opening up your body, as a gardener gently opens up compacted soil.

Appreciate some good things about yourself, remember kind words from other people, and let a warm glow seep through your body. This is like a gardener watering parched soil so plants can grow again.

Now imagine yourself as a plant, with your roots searching for nourishment in this compacted soil. How can you give your roots the resources they need?

Listen for any more ideas and insights. Imagine your body becoming relaxed and dynamic, like healthy earth. Then let your eyes open, and gently come back to here and now.

The term resilience is used a lot for ecosystems — anything from a garden to a whole region. If we look at an ecosystem on a scale we can grasp, like a garden or a farm, we see that its resilience comes from the interweaving of many factors, and we will explore these in later chapters. The concept of ground condition, and how to increase its natural vitality, is a great starting point in deepening the roots of your own human resilience, and measuring progress. Try thinking of yourself as an ecosystem, and keep remembering that all ecosystems (people, farms, gardens) are a natural organism, not a mechanism. This means you can't understand them by mere logic or analysis, and you can't control them. What you can do is understand the best inputs to nourish natural processes, which can be steered towards an outcome you want.

The other common problem in ground condition is *waterlogging*. In soil, this prevents air circulation and damps down fertility. In people, this is like being swamped by feelings, bogged down in emotions. To improve waterlogged soil, you often need a major intervention (like field drains), and the same can be true for waterlogged people: for example, counselling, or a change of circumstances.

How to Nourish Your Ground Condition

Once you start to see yourself as a natural organism, you'll be more aware of what will nourish you, including emotional support, healthy diet, positive physical surroundings. If you listen to your body, it can give you plenty of guidance. The next chapters in this book will show you ways to strengthen your ground condition: including natural energy sources (Chapter 2), and composting (Chapter 3). Get into the habit of strolling around yourself, as a gardener walks round their garden, but with your focus on resources first, and outputs second. Roots before fruits!

Steve's Story: Compaction, Crisis and Cure

Steve asked me for some coaching help. He was 47, a successful software engineer in a personal crisis. His health was going downhill, he was drinking too much, and his wife had threatened to leave unless he sorted himself out. One of the few things they still enjoyed together was gardening.

I briefed Steve on the idea of ground condition, and took him through a self-assessment exercise. Afterwards, he looked worried: 'I can see I'm compacted: in fact, I'm so stuck, I don't know how to change.'

I asked, 'Do you think you take refuge from difficult feelings by working harder?' He groaned. 'Well, yes, but. . .'

I said gently, 'Steve, unless you really cut your work stress, you won't change the compaction, and you won't have space to look at the personal issues.' He nodded. I went on, 'Try imagining that your marriage is like an undernourished tree, with its roots in compacted soil. Can you feel that?'

There was a pause. He sighed deeply. 'It's painful. I've got to open up, give it air, even if it's scary. And I have to work less, and make time to nourish the relationship.'

We agreed some simple steps around exercise, diet and mindfulness to help him relax. I asked him to connect with his own ground condition while he was gardening, to bring the analogy to life. We also agreed that a couples' counsellor would help him to express and hear some difficult feelings, his own and his wife's. After that, the love could start flowing to the roots of the marriage.

A few months later, Steve told me, 'Liz and I both got the likeness between restoring a rundown garden and renewing our relationship. It feels well rooted now. We've been having a weekly check-in to see how we look after the garden of the relationship. '

The Four Stories beneath This Book

This section gives you the gist of my own Story, and of the three projects from which this book has grown: a farm, a garden and a wood.

My Story

My search for happiness grows from unhappy times as a child and teenager. My first answer was to throw myself into work, at school and then in a successful business career. Getting married and being Dad to two wonderful daughters was good, but I still struggled with low self-worth and a need for achievement and reassurance.

In my twenties and thirties I was a happy workaholic: working ridiculous hours and managing businesses in trouble distracted me from deeper issues. By age 40, I realised my job was defining me: so I left the business world, and threw myself into creating an organic farm, hoping to find myself in the process.

Since my early adult years, I've guided my life mostly by intuition and inspiration. Even in my business career, big decisions came this way, not by logic. And since then, I try to stay open to guidance from what I'd call higher wisdom, which can help me serve larger needs, not just my own. I'll explain more about this later in the book.

My forties were a second adolescence. Without a demanding job that defined me, I didn't know who I was. So I explored a lot of meditations and therapies, went travelling, got more insights and more confusion. This led up to the biggest crisis of my life at 49, when my 27-year marriage broke up, I had a cancer scare, and my main consulting client fired me.

My second book, *Out of the Woods*, is about the midlife crisis. I believe midlife may require us to be shipwrecked, dismantled, and reinvent ourselves, and I did it thoroughly. What got me through this crisis were the methods in this book. Living alone for the first time, my garden was my biggest comfort: I learned deeply from it, and from the farm and the wood described below.

Through midlife and beyond, faith in something bigger than the individual has become important: a sense of the Earth as Gaia, living wisdom, plus community connections. I also draw strength from my spiritual path, and believing there's a soul quality that connects all life: this is explored in Chapter 7. I've tried to put my ideals into practice by creating pilot projects which others could learn from and replicate. Two are described below, the others include cohousing neighbourhoods and Seeding our Future, a project helping communities raise resilience to climate change and other issues. See more in Resources below.

One of the ways I've evolved and shared my ideas is through leading workshops. These include many personal development groups and retreats, especially at Magdalen Farm and Hazel Hill Wood, and fascinating work with communities, NHS doctors, social enterprises and businesses on resilience and positive change. All of this has been a rich proving ground for the methods in this book.

Magdalen Farm

I've started several pioneering projects, and have realised that naive ignorance is essential. If you knew a fraction of what you were in for, you'd never begin. In 1990, I had a vision for a project to help kids and teenagers find their feet through contact with Nature. I formed a registered charity and we bought Magdalen Farm in West Dorset.

Magdalen is a 130-acre farm, and we converted it from a rundown beef farm to a certified organic system, with dairy cows, cheese-making, arable crops, pigs and a market garden. Although I had managed some difficult businesses, this was far harder. We were working with animals, plants, weather — natural systems where people aren't in control. That's why listening to the land and the skills of co-creativity, explored in Chapter 4, are so vital.

Starting a mixed organic farm from scratch, and using it as an education centre, meant that I learned the principles and realities of organic farming from the roots up. After 7 years, I realised how this relates to human resilience and sustainability: I started running workshops at the farm, and found that this model worked for other people too. Natural Happiness has grown from these roots.

Our Home Garden

In 2010 my second wife, Linda, and I bought our first house together in Bridport, West Dorset. One appeal of the house was its 1-acre garden, which looked dull, but had potential. The house had been rented out, so it was a low-maintenance garden with lots of lawn, almost no flowers or shrubs, and some overgrown mature trees on the boundaries.

Linda is a keen gardener, who had created gardens in several houses but moved on within a year or two. Here, it was worth investing love, time and money in the garden. I must admit that Linda has more garden expertise than me, but we've learned to share our skills, and go deeper together in listening to the land, and to the spirits of the garden: more on this in Chapter 7.

We're now growing a lot of our own veg and fruit, helped by a polytunnel, greenhouse and fruit cage. Our garden is humming with colour, scent and textures most of the year. We have a wild area at one end, with a retreat cabin for me. There's a lovely sunken garden that we planned together, inspired by Gertrude Jekyll. I've learned that the co-creative approaches of organic farmers are vital for gardeners too. And a garden that you've shaped and nourished gives you back a special kind of happiness and resilience.

Hazel Hill Wood

Hazel Hill Wood is a 70-acre wood near Salisbury. As my daughters entered adolescence, I got interested in vision quests, a Nature immersion process to help teenagers transition towards adult life, and I co-led one at the wood. It was a transformational week for all of us.

I had never spent more than a night at the wood, and had never been there with a group. Suddenly I experienced the wood as a subtle living organism, with a voice that people could tune in to, which had deep wisdom to offer. Slowly, more groups came to the wood, and we created simple, wooden, off-grid buildings, lovingly built by volunteers with a few craftsmen guiding them. We started to combine sustainable forestry with good conservation practices, and the habitat quality and diversity of flowers, birds and other wildlife has improved greatly.

Of the four land-based projects I've started, Hazel Hill is closest to my heart: I've been deeply involved with it for over

30 years. This is a project which has evolved through intuition and inspiration, initially mine, but then with other people too. The decisions about buildings, forestry policy and other matters may not be logical, but I believe those of us steering the project have reached a good level of alignment with the non-human life in the wood.

For many years, I've led groups at the wood helping a wide range of people to explore natural happiness and deepen their resilience. In 2015, I gifted the wood to a new charity, Hazel Hill Trust, and one aim of the expanded project is to continue this work and share it more widely.

Resources

Natural Happiness and Resilience: for blogs and resources, plus information about events with Alan, see **https://www.naturalhappiness.net**. The website includes a guided video version of the tree talk.

Resilience Basics: a good self-help book on the essentials is *Seven Ways to Build Resilience* by Chris Johnstone.

Hazel Hill Wood: for information on events, the project, and a free newsletter, see **https://hazelhill.org.uk**

Cohousing: for more about the two projects Alan initiated see **http://www.thresholdcentre.org.uk** and **https://bridportcohousing.org.uk**

Seeding our Future: this non-profit project helps communities and individuals to raise resilience to climate change and other issues; for example, through skills training and food security projects. See more at **https://www.seedingourfuture.org.uk**

Network of Wellbeing: offers useful events and resources. See **https://networkofwellbeing.org**

Action for Happiness: if you'd like more resources and contacts for local groups on the theme of happiness generally, this may be helpful: see **https://actionforhappiness.org**

Chapter 2

Use Natural Energy Sources

Do you find it's getting harder to find the energy to get through the day? You're not alone! Life and work really are getting more complex and demanding for most of us, so it's no wonder if your energy feels depleted more often.

The earth has an amazing ability to renew its vitality, especially with some human help. We can learn from this, and use natural sources to raise our own energy and resilience. In this chapter, we'll review the four elements of natural energy. We'll also explore how gardening methods, like pruning or crop rotation, can be translated to help you flourish like a healthy ecosystem, and see how to align with the seasonal cultivation cycle.

A gardener uses intuition to 'feel into' what a plant or a bed may need: for example, more light, more water or compost. If you can actually imagine that you're a kind of ecosystem, like a garden, your intuition can guide you about the natural energy sources you need. The earth's vitality is sometimes renewed by activity (such as watering, mulching), sometimes by rest, as in the winter. This is true for people too: and it's better to take such decisions by intuition than by habit. If you're tired from a tough day, a brisk walk may do more to renew you than the glass of wine and soft armchair you usually sink into!

One reason why this topic is so important is that most people face far bigger demands on their personal energy than 10 or 20 years ago. Why is this? One reason is that the average UK person now spends *eight* hours on screens each day (smartphone, computers, TV). Research shows that screen time depletes our energy, and makes it hard to relax fully. Another reason is that social media, the climate crisis, and the sheer pace and complexity of life, all raise our stress levels and drain our energy. And most of us spend less time doing physical work or exercise which could be an antidote.

Natural or Forced Energy Sources?

To explain what natural energy sources mean for people, let's consider the alternative. The differences between organic farming and what's often called industrial or chemical farming can help us clarify the options for human nature.

Conventional farms depend on artificial fertiliser to drive outputs: in effect, plant growth comes mainly from the applied chemicals, not from the vitality of the earth. This promotes rapid but shallow-rooted growth. It pollutes the soil and reduces its fertility. And artificial fertilisers feed problems (weeds and pests) more vigorously than crops. This requires artificial herbicides and pesticides to suppress the problems, causing further pollution to the earth and groundwater. The net result is that the soil and the plants both lack resilience: they become increasingly vulnerable to bad weather, pests and disease. It's a forced energy system, which requires progressively more stimulants and suppressants to make it work, as the diagram shows.

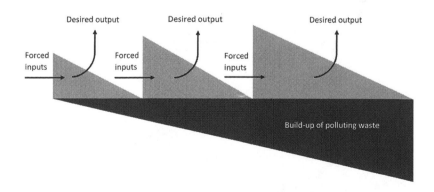

By contrast, organic farms and gardens focus on raising the fertility and resilience of their soil. This takes more effort and time than chemical farming. Compost and manure provide fertility, along with growing 'renewal' crops, also called green manure, like clover which put nitrogen back into the soil. Clever methods to avoid pests include crop rotation, and companion planting, where you use certain plants to attract predators which eat the pests. These approaches avoid the pollution of conventional pesticides.

Can you see the parallels for people? Many people push themselves along on stress, anxiety and caffeine. Social media is another short-term stimulant that depletes us. And many work organisations force outputs through tight deadlines, job insecurity and the gig economy, a culture of fear and competition, and total focus on results. It's easy to get into a habit of suppressing your stress and worries with alcohol, comfort food, gaming and lots more. The consequences of all this are just like forced farming: people lose their natural resilience, become depleted, polluted, and even more dependent on artificial stimulants and suppressants.

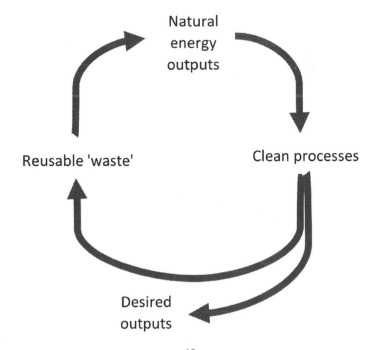

I learned this the hard way, when I got burned out in my early forties after years in high-pressure jobs. So is there a better way to handle living and working under pressure? I've seen natural energy approaches and organic growth methods work for many individuals and groups. There's a limit to how much pressure anyone can handle, but these methods will surely increase your resilience and staying power.

The Four Elements of Natural Energy

How does a gardener get plants to grow? They can't *make* it happen. One crucial part is providing the right kinds of energy: meaning a balanced mix, and clean energy inputs that won't pollute the soil. The same is true for people, but bear with me: explaining how natural energy works for gardens and people is going to get a bit technical.

The analogy between earth and people is a powerful one. A UK expert, Francis Blake, writes in his book *Organic Farming and Growing* that 'the number of micro-organisms (principally bacteria and fungi) in one small teaspoonful of soil is greater than the total number of people who have ever lived on this earth.' The point here is that both people and soil are complex organisms, and we can't expect to understand or manage them in detail.

Instead, what's important is to provide balanced, healthy inputs, have flexible aims about outputs, and let natural processes get on with it. You may remember the four elements viewed by medieval alchemists as the basis of all life: earth, air, fire and water. For gardens and farms, these elements (earth, air, sunlight, water) are the essential growth ingredients, and they give us a simple guide to four energy sources that people need. It's no accident that traditional medicine was often based on these four elements.

Before you read further, I suggest you do the Quickie exercise below. This will help you see how your own ground condition can be improved, and you can try applying the methods in this chapter, instead of reading them as theory.

Self-help Quickie: Listening to Your Land

This process should take 10–15 minutes, though you could spend longer and go deeper. Read these instructions a couple of times, then guide yourself through them from memory if possible.

A gardener listens to the land to know what it needs. In this process, imagine you are the gardener, and your body is the garden. Try to hear the physical needs of your body as a gardener listens to the earth and plants. Here's how.

Take a few long, relaxing breaths. Try to empty your mind of any thoughts or worries. Give your full attention to your physical condition. Scan every part of your body, noticing aches, tensions, and where you feel relaxed or energetic. Imagine all your senses are *inside* your body, so you can hear, touch, see how you are.

Try to imagine your body as a garden: if you're a piece of land, what is your ground condition? Are the plants and trees thriving or struggling? Are you full of vitality, or depleted? Well exercised or tired? Receiving balanced nutrition, or polluted by too much stimulant? What would help?

Now, try listening to your body, as a gardener listens to the land. This may sound odd, but try it, and be patient. You may get an image, or a feeling, or words. Ask your body what it needs. How can you help your body to support you: with more energy, more resilience, more ability to relax?

When you finish, thank your body for what you've learned. Treat it like a friend!

With gardens and farms, we're dealing with physical energy flows. With people, we need to consider both physical and other forms of energy, and how they affect each other. For example, if you're emotionally stressed, this consumes physical energy too, whereas feeling appreciated raises our vitality on all levels. As you explore the four elements in the next section, don't just think about them with your mind, try to feel them in your body. Check how each is for you, and use the analogy with physical elements to assess your energy condition, and what's needed to improve it.

Physical Energy: The Earth Element

The biological activity in the earth is a kind of natural power station. It draws from air, water, sun, waste and minerals. These are converted into fertility: energy for plant growth. Putting this more technically, a balanced set of natural inputs will sustain a high level of organic matter or humus in the soil, and a healthy population of micro-organisms: it's these parts of the soil which are key to its resilience to disease and extreme weather, and to enabling good growth of plants.

The human body is a powerhouse too, if it gets the right energy inputs. For human ground condition our physical inputs, especially food and drink, are a vital influence on our physical energy level. If we rely heavily on kick-start inputs, such as sugary foods and caffeinated drinks, this will create the same problem as artificial fertiliser on the land: the price of the short-term boost is depletion of our underlying vitality. In fact there are strong similarities between the role of microflora in the human gut and in the soil: we can't control them, but we can create the right conditions and diet to help them raise resilience and vitality.

There are many ways to cultivate physical energy: such as aerobic exercise, which gets the circulation moving, and relaxation. Most of us carry stress in our body, which affects physical vitality if it's not released. Everything you do to improve the other three energies will help your physical condition too. If you feel positive, think clearly, and have a strong sense of purpose and vision, imagine how this can raise physical energy — and how the opposite will reduce it.

In cultivating your physical energy, be observant and creative. Many people respond to their physical ailments the way a chemical farmer treats weeds, simply grabbing a quick fix to suppress the symptom. An organic farmer knows that a specific weed has a specific message: it is saying something about the condition of the soil and the response it requires. In the same way, if you know how to observe your physical condition, you can learn what you need to maintain your energy. Complementary health practitioners, such as homeopaths, herbalists, osteopaths or nutritionists, can help you learn this skill.

Emotional Energy: The Water Element

In the growth of the plant and the life of the soil, water has two main functions. First, it carries energy and nutrients down into the earth and up through the plant. Second, the hydrogen and oxygen in water are an energy source in their own right. However, water can also carry problems, such as diseases, or excess nitrates from artificial fertiliser. The system can be parched or swamped: too little or too much water both cause problems.

These properties of water provide pointers for emotional energy in human systems. If I want to move a situation forward, it helps to share positive feelings with others, like appreciation and care. This positive emotional energy will nourish growth, just like watering a plant. Water is a power source in its own right, and so are emotions. For example, appreciation is one of the best natural energisers. Remember a time when you felt deeply valued. Can you recall the flow of energy this created?

Water tends to spread and permeate, so we need to channel it through plumbing and drainage systems. The same is true of emotional energy: we can easily be swamped or flooded by feelings if we don't manage them. We may require a better drainage system: in human terms, this means ways of managing emotions, such as clear communication and conflict resolution (see Chapter 3). We may also need a better balance between the elements. If a piece of ground is waterlogged, air and warmth will help to dry it out. The parallel for people is to engage your sense of purpose and your mental skills to clear an excess of emotion.

Appreciation is a good example of clean energy: renewable and non-polluting. If you feel that your approach to life or work is too dry, what can you do about it? It's quite easy to start a rhythm of appreciation: make a habit of praising more than you criticise. Value yourself and others: this can create a virtuous circle, a progressive spiral in which people around you do the same. In the book *Emotional Intelligence*, Daniel Goleman discusses a number of research studies on how people learn best: it's by feeling recognised and appreciated for what they are doing right, not by being criticised for what they've done wrong.

You may recall how Chapter 1 highlighted compaction and waterlogging as common problems for soil condition, and how these relate to people. Compaction is feeling so uptight that you don't let yourself feel any emotion: the Chapter 1 Self-Help Quickie can help you with this. Waterlogging is feeling swamped by emotion: Chapter 1 covers this too.

Mental Energy: The Fire Element

In this model, fire or sun equates to mental energy. The sun's energy animates the life in the soil and the growth of the plant. In the same way, mental energy enlivens all parts of our life. Mental energy is fiery — and there's more to it than thinking. It includes a flash of intuition, a burst of humour, creativity to spark a new solution, and the burning heat of determined concentration.

Let's dig further into the parallel between sunshine for plants and mental energy for people. In a chilly spring without sun, seeds don't germinate, and there's no growth at all. In a blazing hot summer, plants may get scorched and die. If your brain is cold, inactive, you can't lay plans or make good decisions. And if your brain's on fire, over-active, you may think too much about things, and leave no room for other ways of seeing the situation: for example, the emotional aspects.

You can't force your brain to work: but you can create the right conditions, give it stimulus, and steer it. Research shows that mental energy is stronger when you're physically healthy and relaxed, when you have variety and a sense of purpose in your life, and when you're neither repressed nor swamped emotionally.

If you really imagine mental energy as fire, this should give you guidelines for generating and managing mental energy. I find it helpful to picture my brain like a wood-burning stove. If the fuel is too wet, it's hard to start the fire, and I get choking smoke instead of useful heat. Conversely, if the wood is too dry, I get high heat for a while but no sustained output. We often think of emotion as impeding our brain, which it does at the extremes. However, the most productive mix, for plant and human growth, is moderate amounts of both heat and water. Used well, emotional energy can fuel our mental processes and raise our overall effectiveness: so nourishing our wellbeing, feeling happy, helps us think more clearly!

Fire also needs air for combustion. To get a stove started and burning strongly, I need to open the stove's dampers wide and provide plenty of air. And to kill the flame, all I have to do is shut off the air flow. This highlights the connection between mental and inspirational energy. To fire up your mind, you need a strong sense of purpose and vision. When life feels pointless, our brain shuts down.

Inspirational Energy: The Air Element

For plant growth, air has two key functions. First, as an enabler: healthy soil has around 25 per cent air content, and these spaces let water, warmth and air circulate within the earth to generate growth. Secondly, the air is a source of fertility: 78 per cent of our atmosphere is nitrogen.

The air element equates to inspirational energy: a sense of higher purpose, wider perspective and vision. The term inspiration, like the word spirit, derives from the Latin *spiritus*, meaning breath, air or soul. What this model highlights is that vision and purpose are a powerful energy source, a fuel for growth in their own right. Think about outstanding achievement in any field: sport, the arts, service to society, or your own life. Inspiration is part of the power we need for real fulfilment.

Consider the qualities of air, and how these also describe inspirational energy. It's invisible, intangible, yet always around us, available. If we are tense or defensive, our breath is shallow and we don't access its full potential. There's a link between inspiration and breath: if I am tense, taking several long, slow breaths gives me a sense of expansion and relaxation, helping me to see the situation in perspective and connect with my intention and purpose. Breathing more deeply adds oxygen to the bloodstream, which enhances brain activity and mental energy. It also helps to release physical and emotional stress.

Accessing your inspirational energy can be as easy as breathing, but other techniques are also important. Find a visioning process which works for you, which enables you to find clarity and purpose even in complex and confusing situations: this is explored in Chapter 7, along with other ways to access inspiration. You may need to cultivate your ground condition and soil structure to be able to harness the air element. For example, compacted or waterlogged soil and people all need more air.

Personal Energy Management

Gardeners and farmers manage the energy mix for their land, and you can do this for your personal ecosystem. The four types of human energy we've just explored give you a framework for understanding and improving your natural energy flows. Checking your ground condition, including the four energy elements, can be a quick and helpful approach. Imagine yourself as a garden to bring this all to life. Using practical images (earth – physical, water – emotional, fire – mental, air – inspirational) should give you specific pointers on how to manage your energy use, and access more vitality when you need it.

One of the tools I've developed is a Personal Energy Audit, to help you understand where your energy comes from, where you use it, and how to raise your vitality level. This parallels the way gardeners and farmers use soil tests to show them how to improve fertility, and what plants or crops will grow best. The Personal Energy Audit helps you assess four types of energy: physical, emotional, mental and inspirational. You'll find this in the Appendix.

Case History: Janine's Personal Energy Audit

When Janine came on one of my Natural Happiness workshops, she told us, 'I'm desperate: I'm so stressed and burned out I can't take any more. I work as an office manager in a busy insurance broker — my boss, who owns the business, is a bully. He only cares about results. I'm a

---

natural worrier, so he winds me up constantly, I can't stop fretting about my work.'

When Janine did the Personal Energy Audit, here are the main things she learned:

- 'I'm depending on unhealthy food and drink as a major energy inflow, but I realise it's a major outflow too, because the buzz wears off quickly and it leaves me depleted.'
- 'My work is a massive emotional outflow, and I'm leaning heavily on family and friends for support, which is unhealthy for everyone, and so unfair on my kids.'
- 'Because I'm so anxious, I waste mental energy fretting, and I can't find creative ways to improve my situation.'
- 'There's almost no inspirational energy flowing in any part of my life. Doing the Audit has helped me realise I'm actually depressed: not only does my work feel pointless, so does everything else, which is really painful.'

Approaching this like a gardener helped Janine to see how she could change things. Her first priority was her physical ground condition: both exercising and relaxing outdoors helped her stop her dependency on junk food and coffee. She also realised she was compacted: too tense to compost her stress, or to let in support. Her changes in physical energy helped, and she got some counselling help.

At first Janine was sure she should quit her job. But she decided to face up to her boss. She explained how stressed she was, and said she'd have to leave unless she could change the way she worked. Janine asked her boss to let her do things her way for a 3-month trial, including guidelines on how and when the boss communicated with her.

Janine had assessed the ground condition of her team, and during the 3 months ran weekly sessions where she and her team could appreciate and support each other. Janine told me, 'The high-pressure, results-only atmosphere my boss created was hard for all of us. I realised we were all desperate for some kindness and appreciation, not just me. So, when I started to express this, I really did create an upward spiral.'

She had to assert herself to hold her boss to the guidelines. At the 3-month review, Janine and her boss agreed it was working: staff absences and turnover were down, clients were happier, and the renewal rate had improved.

Janine said, 'Another benefit of being more fit and relaxed physically was that my sense of purpose and perspective returned. I know why I'm doing the job, and it doesn't dominate my whole life anymore.'

Depletion and Regeneration

Worldwide, millions of acres of farmland are in a state of ongoing depletion, their fertility and resilience exhausted by years of chemical farming. It's probably fair to say that there are millions of people in ongoing depletion too. Living with high levels of uncertainty, and an overload of worrying news, is inherently exhausting.

One of the exciting recent trends in farming is regenerative agriculture. This involves methods that not only sustain resilience and fertility, but aim to increase it and protect it in the face of challenges like climate change. Many experts also believe that farms could adapt their methods to sequester large volumes of CO_2 from the atmosphere: for more on this, see Charles Eisenstein's book in Resources.

If you feel systematically depleted, imagine you can create a plan for your own regeneration. All the tools are in this book. Here are some pointers:

- Do the Personal Energy Audit, identify what drains your energy, what raises it, and change your ways of living and working to shift the balance.
- In regenerative agriculture, specific crops can be grown to open up compacted soil, raise fertility and so on. Look for your equivalents, such as counselling, creative hobbies, a project that truly inspires you, or a supportive friendship.
- A fallow or rest period is used on farms converting to organic methods: you may need some fallow time too.
- A key element in regenerative farming is de-intensification: this means reducing your output goals, putting less demands on your land, so you don't need chemical inputs. For us humans, downshifting can do the same.
- When an organism stops being dosed with artificial stimulants and suppressants, there's usually a period of turbulence: you may need to prepare yourself and people around you for a mix of exhaustion, buried emotions arising, cravings and bewilderment. A strong vision of how you want to be is a good counterweight.
- Regenerative methods require more skill and patience than depleting ones: you need to find the time and commitment to invest in learning and sticking with a new approach.
- You will probably need to drop some habits and dependencies to make this change: setting a vision and a plan, and asking a few of your family and friends to support you, can help.

Gardening Skills to Help Your Personal Ecosytem

Seeing yourself as an ecosystem is just a more technical version of cultivating yourself like a garden. By using natural systems ideas, like the Personal Energy Audit, we can bring deeper understanding and better techniques to looking after ourselves. In this section, we'll explore how a range of gardening methods can be translated for human use.

When a gardener sets priorities for their garden, observation and reflection are essential, whether they're planning today's work or a whole year's programme. Walking the land, noticing, sitting to reflect, giving space for intuition: all these are basic for gardeners, farmers, and for you with your personal ecosystem. Sometimes I ask people to make a drawing of themselves as a garden or a farm, to imagine aspects of themselves like a vegetable plot, a flock of sheep or chickens, or an orchard: the more you can bring this analogy to life for yourself, the more it can help you. So, as you read about these gardening methods, see yourself as both the garden and the gardener.

Pruning: Cut Back to Grow Forward

In our society, cutbacks always sound like something bad. But if you're shaping natural growth, cutting and pruning are vital skills. Pruning plants is done for various purposes: such as boosting growth generally, or getting more of an output you want (such as flowers or fruit), or to maintain health by removing diseased areas and letting air circulate.

Pruning is a complex blend of art and science. The technique and time of year will vary by the plant and the reason for pruning. Cutting into plants, especially bigger shrubs and trees, can be scary. But as Monty Don says, 'You shouldn't be afraid of it, because plants have an inbuilt system of regrowth in response to damage — and all pruning is a form of damage, as far as plants are concerned. With astonishingly simple but delicate control, every tree or shrub regulates its own growth according to the size of its branches and the extent of its roots.'

As you'll recall from Chapter 1, this balance of roots, branches and fruits is important for people too, so we need the courage and skills to cut back on ourselves sometimes. The first step, as in the garden, is to be clear what you want more or less of. Then plan what, when and how to cut. Here are some examples from people on my workshops: names and details disguised:

- Neera realised that one group of friends were pulling her into bitchiness and bingeing, and she gradually withdrew from them.
- Nick worked out that his full-time job was actually taking 60 hours a week: he asked to cut back his responsibilities, and to move to 4 days a week.
- Natalie and Paul were exhausted by caring for Paul's father, and saw that they had to reduce their time for this, and seek more help.
- Pat complained of exhaustion, but then realised her smartphone was on for 14 hours a day: cutting this to 6 hours gave some rest and renewal space.

In a human sense, pruning can be less sudden and irreversible than for plants. We can consult, negotiate, experiment about the cuts we feel we need, and even reduce or reverse the changes we've made.

Mulching: Snuggle into TLC

In organic gardens, mulching is a key way to avoid chemical weed treatment and fertiliser. A mulch is typically a layer of compost, bark, grass cuttings, or a mix of all three, spread over a bed or around each plant. It has several benefits:

- It keeps moisture in the soil

- It suppresses weeds by natural means
- It improves soil fertility and plant growth

In Chapter 3, we'll explore what composting means for land and people. In gardens, one of the main ways compost is used to help fertility is by mulching. Young plants are vulnerable, and weeds can crowd them out: putting mulch around the crop you want suppresses the weeds which might compete with them. As spring turns to summer, full growth needs moisture and nutrition. For human nature, mulching means heaping up resources, creating reserves, giving yourself some TLC and protection. Here are some examples:

- When Angie got a promotion, she planned some evenings with friends and quiet weekends away, to give her extra nourishment in the first 6 months.
- Bruce and Sue moved back in together, after a painful 6-month separation. Couples counselling had helped them to compost the anger and blame, and they made a commitment to care for each other, handle conflicts cleanly, and have some fun. One evening a week would be a mutual mulching session!
- Steve was easily distracted, spending hours on social media, and he realised this was like weeds competing with the plants he wanted to grow. His mulching was to create regular habits, like jogging and mindfulness, which filled the spaces.

Crop Rotation: Growing through Rest and Renewal

Crop rotation is one of my favourite cycles, and one that I use several times a week. In vegetable gardens and organic farms, crop rotation is a natural means of sustaining fertility and reducing weeds and pests. It means that a variety of crops are grown in different years on the same piece of land. Often these will include a renewal crop, which rebuilds fertility after a demanding one. Or sometimes the land will be left fallow and rested for a season.

If you grow the same crop on the same land, year after year, this will attract more pests and weeds. Varying the crop reduces these problems. Large industrial farms will devote hundreds of acres to one crop for years, and need heavy use of pesticides and herbicides because of this. Often, it's the most valuable crops that demand most from the soil, such as wheat. At Magdalen Farm, 3 years of growing wheat on a field were followed by 2 years growing clover, which naturally replaces nitrogen in the soil.

Use Crop Rotation to Sustain Your Energy

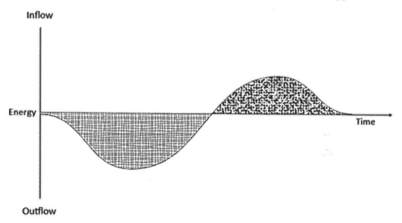

Follow an energy-demanding activity with a renewing one, like a walk, a break, a chat with a friend

The benefits of crop rotation for your personal ecosystem, or a group, can be similar. Consciously try to vary your activities; for example, between solitary and sociable, analytical and creative. When I've just finished a demanding task, I do something restorative, like go for a walk, or phone a friend for a chat. If your work tasks are all similar, this may be depleting you, so look for ways to bring some variety in. This could also be true for your home or leisure life. Use the Personal Energy Audit to see where more variety could increase your energy inflows and minimise losses.

Progressing in Cycles: The Four Seasons

We live in a society that thinks all progress is linear: forward and upward is good, but going round in circles must be bad. Anyone who works with the land knows that natural growth moves in cycles, and it's true for human nature too. The seasons of the year shape everything a gardener does, and they're a great guide for your life and work.

Many people are in continual spring and summer: they're constantly starting and pushing things, and never make time for harvesting, maintaining, rest and review: the autumn and winter seasons. Other people may be stuck in a winter phase of lethargy. The benefit of mapping yourself with the four seasons is to see which phases of the cycle you neglect or overdo: balancing your seasons will improve your resilience and your enjoyment of life. The Cultivation Cycle Checklist later in this chapter will help you to do this.

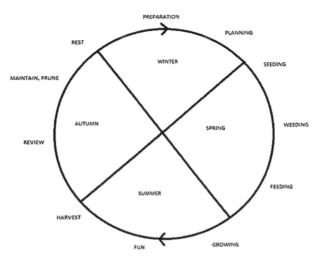

Cultivation cycle: the four seasons

Although the four seasons on the land are an annual cycle, you personally will need to move through these seasons more often. To some extent, you need them all daily, weekly and monthly. Even in the garden, each season isn't exactly 3 months long, and activities don't always align with the cycle of the calendar year. For instance, some crops are sown in autumn and harvested in spring. You will probably find that aspects of your life and work are at different stages of this cycle.

The four seasons model might imply that each season should be of equal length, but for people this is hardly realistic, and the autumn and winter phases are likely to be squeezed. One crucial aspect of these more receptive seasons is quiet time, when you can rebuild resources and deeper understanding can emerge as the groundwork and seed for the next turn of the cycle. Let's look at each season more closely.

Winter: Preparation

In the cultivation cycle, each season is a prelude to the next. The winter period of rest and review creates the platform for spring growth. Soil is largely dormant: this helps build the energy reserves for the intense growth ahead. This is also the time when a gardener reviews ground condition, adds compost, and plans the spring plantings.

For people, this is the season for rest, renewal and preparation. Even a short downtime — a pause for stillness, reflection, and perspective — can be helpful. It's a stage in the cycle where you should review and renew your ground condition: improving structure, mixing in compost, so that you are ready for the coming growth season. This is also a time for planning your crops, looking ahead through the whole cycle to prepare for it: setting your goals, making a schedule, identifying skills, support or resources you need.

Spring: The Delicate Start

Seeding and establishing plants in the garden is a time of intense human activity. Getting the growth process started is the most delicate stage. New seeds are vulnerable: if the soil is too cold or too dry, the seed won't germinate, and the process of growth won't even begin. If the ground is too wet, the seed will rot instead of grow. In this early phase, the plants are vulnerable to weather extremes, such as frost: close attention and quick response can bring the young crop through; for example, applying a layer of fleece to protect it. The right conditions for seeding the desired plants will also stimulate the weeds. Slow-growing crops risk being out-competed for resources by weeds, which are often vigorous and fast growing. Hence this period of early growth is the busiest time for weeding as well as seeding and feeding. Fast-growing, nutrient-hungry crops such as tomatoes may need extra help.

Does this have parallels for you? Starting a new friendship, or a new project, is more like cultivating a plant than turning on a computer. Your success rate and speed of progress will improve if you give plentiful attention to this season: preparing the ground, providing a balanced supply of the four growth elements, protecting the new crop, staying observant and dealing with problems as they arise. Watering is especially important: nourishing the new starts with love and appreciation. Beginnings can lead to misunderstandings, mistakes, unexpected outcomes: this is why the observation and patience of weeding is needed. And recognise that this season demands a lot of resources, so reduce other demands on your energy, and line up as much support for yourself as you can.

Summer: Letting It Roll

One lesson of the summer season is to know when to stop pushing and allow natural growth to get on with it. However, for some crops further management may be needed: hoeing out weeds or thinning the crop so that the strongest plants can reach their full potential. For people, it's a season to let your energy flow productively, along with fun and relaxation. It's also a time to celebrate your progress. The Celtic festival of Lammas around August 1 was the start of giving thanks for the year's produce, and it's a good approach throughout your life and work.

Autumn: The Harvest

Harvesting, gathering in the completed crop, lasts through summer into autumn. There may be several stages in moving from the crop to the finished product. Consider wheat: once the plant is cut, the grain must be separated from the husk and the stalk, then dried before further processing. Similarly, in your life allow time to harvest the full value and nutrition from your outputs.

Autumn brings us to completion of the gathering-in phase, and the season of harvest festival. Appreciating and celebrating the fruits of the earth and our labour is another basic element in the cycle. Then, as plant growth slows right down, we move into gathering our stores: preparing for winter. It's also a time for pruning, cutting back old growth to improve the coming year's production, seeing what maintenance and renewal are required.

For people, the autumn season is vital in making the growth cycle sustainable as well as productive. This is the time for reviewing and learning, tending and regenerating your production capacity. This is also where you get the full fruits of your crop: through learning, celebration, and knowing how to process and store some of the output. You need to gather up appreciation and insights to give you energy through your own winter periods. Without this, you risk getting only superficial benefits from the whole growth cycle.

The Cultivation Cycle Checklist

Each stage of the cultivation cycle is important. Most of us tend to focus on a few stages of this cycle, and neglect others. This checklist can also be helpful in looking at how a whole group approaches things, such as a work team or community organisation.

Give each item a rating from 0 – total neglect, through 5 – balance, to 10 – major overemphasis.

CYCLE STAGE	YOUR RATING
Ground preparation: planning, nurturing the starting phase	
Seeding: using creativity	
Weeding: learning through problems, maintaining clarity	
Feeding: raising momentum by support, vision, and appreciation	
Fun: enjoying, celebrating, enabling enthusiasm to produce growth	
Harvesting: completion, reaping full benefits, storing the fruits	
Review: drawing out the learning and appreciating people	...
Maintaining: preparing/renewing/pruning for future growth	
Rest: yes, rest!	

Use this checklist to appreciate the stages in the cycle which you or a group do well, and to highlight stages where you would benefit from more attention.

Resources

Personal Energy Audit: You'll find this in the Appendix.

If the gardening analogy appeals to you, you can explore it further by reading gardening books, and imagining the human parallels. Here are some which are especially relevant:

The Complete Gardener, by Monty Don. This is a best-selling book on organic gardening. Monty combines huge experience with a delightful style of writing, and a good sense of wider implications.

Bob Flowerdew's *Organic Gardening Bible*. Bob is a leading UK expert on organic gardening. His first chapter, The Organic Way, has a lot of human parallels.

Organic Gardening: The Natural no-dig Way, by Charles Dowding. A readable practical guide, mainly for vegetable and fruit growing, which can help you see the human parallels.

Hidden Nature, by Alys Fowler: a deep exploration of connections between Nature around us and within us.

Permaculture: this is a systemic approach to integrating humans and Nature in gardening, and in society generally. You can get the gist at **https://permacultureprinciples.com**. And I highly recommend Permaculture Magazine: see **https://www.permaculture.co.uk**

Climate, a new story, by Charles Eisenstein. If you want a well-researched overview about regenerative agriculture, with examples of what it could contribute to carbon sequestration, Chapter 8 provides it.

Chapter 3

Compost Your Troubles

Imagine you can harness a major source of energy, that's already within you: it's free, abundant, and just needs a bit of effort to process it. What's more, you'll be creating benefits out of problems that drain energy and pollute your inner ecosystem. This is what composting offers you.

In this chapter, we'll explore in detail how composting works in the garden, how it can work for you, and how it can help groups and teams. You'll also find pointers on techniques to help you compost difficult situations with other people: creative conflict resolution and natural communication. And you can learn how 'changing the Story' can compost a repeating pattern of negative feelings.

In a natural system, there is no waste. Composting in gardens and farms starts with rubbish, animal dung, rotting vegetable matter. All this 'waste', useless in these forms, ends up as humus, highly fertile, able to renew the earth's vitality. Now imagine the waste that's stuck in your ecosystem: emotions, mental worry, maybe a sense of pointlessness. And feel how great it would be to clear out this waste and turn it into fresh energy and insights. Consider how much of your energy is tied up in negative emotions like anger, or in anxious thoughts and mental stress. Composting can help you turn all this into positive energy and insights, but it's a new skill which takes patience. In this chapter, you will find several ways to put composting into practice, and ways to use it with other people.

Composting waste in the garden raises the vitality and resilience of your soil, and avoids the pollution and depletion caused by artificial fertiliser. Physical composting takes several months but the human equivalent can happen in minutes, days or weeks. Plant and animal waste usually look bad, and smell worse. Yet they are a valuable resource if we can change their form, and the same is true of human energy waste.

Human Energy Waste

By human energy waste, I don't mean car exhaust fumes or old plastic cups: I mean personal energy that's stuck or stagnant in a negative form. Here are some examples:

Physical: stress and toxins that build up in your body, due to anxiety, unhealthy food and drink, etc.

Emotional: negative feelings like anger or depression, and unresolved conflicts.

Mental: habitual worrying, going round in circles in your mind, about big issues or everyday ones.

Inspirational: a sense of hopelessness or pointlessness about aspects of your own life and work, or the state of the world.

Most of us carry a lot of negative energy, stuck in our ecosystem, which saps our vitality. The first two steps are noticing it, and making moves to compost some of this into a source of positive energy.

Composting in Action

There are three levels of composting you can use:

- **In the moment:** Try using the Quickie process below as soon as you feel upset. If someone just said something to cause this, slow the situation down: ask them to repeat it, or say 'Give me a minute to digest that.'
- **Review and reflect:** A good way to maintain your resilience is by a regular review of anything that's bugging you and

sapping your energy. For this, the Seven Steps process is worth using. To do this thoroughly, you may need to intensify difficult feelings, so find a space and time where you can complete the composting.

- **Professional help:** if you're facing a major upset in your personal life or your work, it may be wise to get support from a counsellor or therapist. Part of their training is in composting painful emotions, though they may not use this language.

The Quickie process below is worth memorising, so you can use it in real time when something upsets you.

Self-help Quickie: Short Composting Process

Use this while you're in an upsetting situation, or when you don't have much time to deal with a difficult feeling.

Start by focussing your attention in your body. Feel the weight of your feet on the floor. Look for any physical signs of tension, take note of them (such as shallow breathing, sweaty palms).

Now start breathing slowly and deeply: push on the outbreath, so you empty your lungs. Imagine you are moving your breath and your attention around your body in a circular flow, starting from where you feel most distress. See yourself breathing the difficult feelings up your spine to your head, then down the front of your body to the perineum.

As you continue this circular breathing, imagine you are converting your distress into clean, positive energy.

With practice, you can do this for a minute or two while you're in a challenging situation. Or use it soon afterwards.

From Gardens to Humans: A Seven Step Composting Guide

Gardeners use a range of composting techniques: these seven steps are based on hot aerobic composting, because it has the best parallels for people. Before you apply this, read all seven steps, and you may find the case study useful. To build up your capacity, I suggest you start by using this process for relatively smaller issues, and build up from there.

1. **Gathering your rubbish**

   Your first step is to identify and gather some of the waste in your life and work. This may include difficult feelings and festering situations that smell nasty: you might rather bury them, but stick with it! Start with **physical waste**, reviewing tensions in your body, and health issues. Then consider **mental waste**: nagging problems, unresolved puzzles.

   Next, gather the **emotional waste**, identifying feelings you're upset by. Identify the sources, such as particular situations or relationships. Keep breathing as you do this, aerating the compost. Name and explore feelings such as fear, anxiety, uncertainty, anger. Use as much mental clarity as you can to understand the causes. Think of these waste feelings as a flow of energy that is stuck, and see what outcome would unblock them.

   Negative **inspirational energy** can be the most depleting and difficult to face. A sense of pointlessness is like a major pollution problem: pervasive and hard to clear. Use the parallel: it can arise from one main source like a dirty factory, or from a diffuse problem like road traffic. Either way, a systemic change is probably needed: a switch to clean energy sources and processes, and more recycling. Imagine what that would mean for you.

In counselling it is often said that expressing a problem is already halfway to resolving it. Gathering and identifying your waste issues is a big step forward in the recycling process. And avoid judging yourself or the issue as far as possible.

2. **Sorting and heaping**

If you've done your gathering thoroughly, by now you may be feeling rather daunted and overwhelmed. The sorting stage should help. In garden composting, you don't put all waste on the heap: some stuff is hard to break down, or simply unsuitable. When you start on human energy composting, build up your skills and confidence by starting on smaller, easier issues, and getting some early wins. Typically, physical and mental issues are easier to compost than emotional or inspirational ones. Some issues may be so big that you need professional help.

Compost needs to be heaped up, so that there is a critical mass of material for the biological processes to start. It may feel risky to let your issues intensify, but try it. You build your compost heap by facing your waste issues fully and deeply: just allow the feelings, observe them, and don't deny or judge them. Keep your sense of purpose and perspective: remember that you are more than your feelings. And ensure that you have support available.

3. **Air supply**

Air fuels the biological activity in the composting process. For you, this means that when you feel strong emotions, keep breathing! And affirm your sense of purpose: you need inspirational energy to fuel this transformation. Deeper breathing is a classic way to stay steady amid difficult feelings, and mindfulness methods can also help.

4. **Water content**

The ideal moisture content in a compost heap is around 50 per cent. Relating this to human energy, if you are too dry and you deny or repress your feelings, recycling is stifled. Exploring the issues with a friend or counsellor may give you the encouragement and sense of safety to let them flow. Conversely, if you are swamped by your feelings and the compost heap is sodden, the waste will fester, not transform. In this situation, your compost needs more heat and air: mental clarity, and a sense of perspective and connection to the bigger picture.

5. **Heat**

High temperature is central to this process of transforming muck into gold. Micro-organisms combine with air and moisture to generate heat from decomposing the waste, and the heat usefully kills weed seeds and pathogens. For people, composting should generate heat, mental energy, which can then take the process further. You should find that composting your waste issues generates fresh understanding, clear thinking to move you forward.

6. **Turning**

To get the full benefit of the composting process, it is common to turn the heap after a few weeks. This means inverting the compost to aerate it. Turning the compost heap increases the air supply and renews the recycling process: the effect is to achieve fuller breakdown of the waste, and generate higher humus content.

You may find that composting your own energy waste takes anything from minutes to months: in human terms, turning your compost means reviewing your progress, and linking what may be a difficult process of recycling to a bigger sense of purpose. When you remind yourself this is about feeling happier and re-energised, clearing obstacles that have held you back, it should help you persist. Aeration is about connecting to your inspiration and the bigger picture.

My experience of human energy composting is that the process is largely self-directing and has its own momentum. It sometimes may be tiring and distressing, but trust it. Periodically I'm aware of this process going on within me and give it my attention, but I don't have to make it happen.

7. **Application**

So you've got your compost: how will you use it? Consider your priorities as you start to gain energy from your composting process. If your ground condition is depleted, limit your activities, and feed the essential ones. If you have one demanding challenge, focus your new resources on it. You can also use your Personal Energy Audit from Chapter 2 to guide you.

Composting Case Study: Marion's Storm

I'm including this case study to show you how composting can work in practice.

Financial Friends was a small coaching client: Phil and Marion Wood had started this business while they were married, and set it up as a formal partnership when they divorced. Their business was financial advice, selling pension plans and life insurance.

In ground condition terms, Phil was waterlogged, Marion was dry and hard as rock. I suggested an individual session for me with each of them.

Beneath Marion's hard crust of logical criticism, I suspected she had buried a lot of feelings about the marriage and the business partnership with Phil. I took my usual 'park and ride' approach: using my conscious mind to clarify the question, and leaving my subconscious to come up with an answer. That afternoon, driving through sultry June weather, I began to think about thunderstorms and I started laughing: this image gave me an approach with Marion.

Stoking Up a Storm

When we met, we piled up observations on the problems of the business. She was getting increasingly tense and heated as the issues were heaped together. I sought to step up the heat by piling the waste higher, voicing my own emotions about it. I made a link to the air element and the overall vision of the business.

'Marion,' I said, 'I feel really upset by all these concerns you are listing. These are major problems, serious. . .'

'Very serious.' Marion was twisting her hand as she spoke.

'What also really upsets me, Marion, is how this affects you. I can't imagine how you're feeling. . .'

'Feeling!' The storm broke. She leapt to her feet, shouting, picked up the vase from her dining table and threw it so hard that it shattered on the wall. 'Feeling! I want to kill him! How can I get it right with a man like that?'

For some time, Marion stormed on, alternating between rage at Phil and weeping with a pent-up mixture of sadness, pain and frustration. Remembering how the heat needs to rise in the early stage of composting, I urged her to let the feelings flow instead of trying to calm her down.

As Marion became quieter, I raised questions about purpose and perspective, to aerate and turn the compost. 'Do you still have a sense of vision for Financial Friends?'

I asked her. 'How would you like to see the business develop from here?'

These questions certainly renewed the composting process. I was impressed that Marion was already combining feelings, thoughts and perspective. 'Alan, the point is, Financial Friends is Phil and me. You can't have a vision for this business without having a vision of how the two of us relate. That's what I feel desperate about.'

'Desperate?'

'Well, desperate in my confusion. I have this sense that we have negative patterns between us, going back years, and it's exhausted us. But what I can't see is, could both of us change enough to make it work properly?'

Turning the Compost

Marion started pacing restlessly around the room. I took this as a good sign that her energy was getting moving. 'It's always been like this with Phil. I try to do my part perfectly. Then if there's any problem, it must be his fault.'

I nodded. 'So how do you feel toward him now?'

She clenched her fists. 'Angry! Oh yes, angry. Bloody furious, in fact.'

I stood up, and came closer to her. 'So, what I suggest is, intensify the feeling. Picture scenes that upset you, remember how the business is suffering, and feel your fury. Speak to him. Do you want to pick an object to represent him?'

Marion smiled. 'OK. The television set can be Phil. I'll get as good a hearing from the telly as I would from him.'

She kept pacing the room, and I could see the tension rising in her body, until at last she started shouting. As the raw rage passed, the fertile insight that emerged was: 'I can't achieve anything except through you, Phil.'

At this point, I intervened. 'So, you're still furious, but now you can see why. Right?'

She nodded. 'Right.'

'Keep feeling the fury, and ask yourself a question. Forget Phil: What would you like to do with this anger? You've got this terrific energy you've unleashed: How do you want to use it? Imagine that you can achieve things without him. What do you want to achieve? Keep walking, keep feeling the anger, but breathe it, circulate it.'

She looked puzzled. 'What do you mean, circulate it?'

I came over and stood next to her. 'So you're angry: where in your body do you feel it?'

She held her stomach. 'Here. Definitely.'

'OK. So, imagine breathing this anger up your spine, through your brain, down to your heart, and back to your stomach. Think of the anger like steam: it's scalding, but there's a power you can harness. Picture these questions like the pistons in a steam engine: you feed the anger in, and you can get forward motion out.'

There was a long silence. Marion walked slowly around the room. I could actually watch the cycle of her breathing in, moving the anger up, then releasing the energy to continue the cycle. After a while she sat down. Eventually she opened her eyes and smiled at me. 'This is such a relief,' she said. 'I've got past blaming someone else. I can see that I'm quite capable. I'm not good at handling clients, but I don't have to depend on Phil for it. We could bring in a second sales consultant, and I can channel the leads through them.'

This intense composting session left Marion with fresh energy and clarity. I had a very different session with Phil, helping drain some of his swamping emotions. I then guided a session with both of them using conflict resolution methods.

Composting, Conflict, Communication

Many of the issues we need to compost involve our connection with other people. What can we learn from gardens to do it better? In an ecosystem, what seems like waste or loss is a gain or nutrient for some other part of the system. For a better approach to conflict and competition between people, look at the whole system, and where there's a flow of benefits even in situations that look negative.

In the natural world, animals or plants that compete with each other will collaborate at other times. If you feel stuck in an adversarial position, try to compost the feelings so you can see when there's scope for cooperation. There are also useful skills you may already have as a gardener: deep connection with Nature brings *humility*: you can't fully understand or control this system, so you know your limitations. And it brings *integrity*: roots in the realities of the situation, and in fundamental principles, not in ego or imaginings. As a gardener, you know you need patience, observation, careful exploring, when you meet a challenge. All this helps our dealings with other people too.

You may feel that in this section we're a long way from gardening skills, but that's only partly true. If you can approach conflict and communication problems with a gardener's mindset, it will help. This is not just the skills in the paragraph above: it's also seeing yourself and other people as organisms, not mechanisms. You can influence them and co-create with them (as explored in the next chapter), you can't control them or force them to the outcome you'd like. Human skills which can help you to compost difficult situations include conflict resolution and natural communication.

Creative Conflict Resolution

We often regard conflicts as bad, but they're a normal part of life in the human and natural worlds. Many people find conflicts alarming, and react in fight-or-flight mode: conflicts are hot situations and need careful handling to avoid someone being hurt. The three-stage process summarised below is drawn from experts in conflict management: for a full version of this process, see Resources.

Conflict brings up strong emotions, and people can move quickly from the facts of the present situation into a habit or pattern. This can mean getting angry and aggressive, or walking away and cutting off, or going quiet and not expressing their views. Sometimes you can use these three stages quickly and simply. In more serious situations, it helps to have more time, and some independent support.

Stage 1: Cooling. Many conflicts heat up and escalate very quickly. This stage aims to prevent or quickly redress this, with three main steps:

- Hear the other party's feelings
- Slow the process down
- Restore respect

Stage 2: Clarifying. This stage begins when both parties' emotional heat has reduced to a level where they can talk about how to proceed from here, and about the issues and needs they have. A third-party mediator will make this much easier. The clarifying stage has four aims:

- To deal with any power and safety issues that could prevent true negotiation
- To form an initial agreement on a process to resolve the conflict
- To get all the needs and issues out on the table and understood by both parties
- To develop an atmosphere of trust, safety and collaboration as a basis for the third stage

Stage 3: Construction. The aim in this stage is for the parties to work together to construct a satisfactory solution. This stage can begin once all the aims of the clarifying phase are fulfilled. The methods could include:

- Highlight the bigger picture of the whole relationship and its benefits
- Focus on a solution to serve future needs, not resolving all the historic problems
- Use composting methods

Conflict Resolution Case Study: The Odd Couple

Steve and James had been in partnership for 8 years, as small-scale, upmarket property developers. They'd always struck me as an unlikely mix: Steve a sweaty, no-nonsense builder, and James cool, smartly dressed, the architect and front man. Now the relationship had broken down, and they asked me to help them clear the air and negotiate a severance deal.

Neither of them was good at expressing feelings, so the Cooling Stage had to rely a lot on grunts and nods. I did establish that neither of them felt respected by the other: I used a tactic from marriage guidance, and asked them to recall what they liked about each other when they first got together. That got them smiling, and meant they could start a conversation.

In the clarifying stage, it was soon clear that there was a major power and safety issue, for both of them. James felt upset because Steve had all the company assets in his name. Steve felt James was so clever he'd pull tricks on him. We unpacked this, exploring 'the worst that could happen'.

I asked them to recollect times they'd helped each other through a crisis, and got them to assure each other they wouldn't take advantage. By now they could both see that a written separation agreement would help.

I asked both of them to say what was most important in the outcome of this breakup. That took trust from both of them, but it brought in a quality of collaboration. I was touched that both of them said maintaining mutual liking and respect was their top concern. We looked at why their partnership had broken down, and cleared up some misunderstandings. We also agreed on timings for two more meetings, so they had a structure to work within.

As I prepared for the first meeting of the Construction Phase, I could see that both Steve and James felt like losers, and had no confidence they could handle this situation. It was painful to see two successful entrepreneurs with their tails down. And then I thought: these guys are experts in construction!

So, I asked them to treat this breakup agreement like a proposal for a housing project. What are the outcomes, what are the problems, how's it going to be viable? They perked up at once. We actually assigned different parts of the 'proposal' to each of them, and started to put a draft together.

I knew we hadn't fully resolved the hurt feelings, but believed we'd get a working solution by focussing on the practical level, with an honest dialogue about what they both needed. They were happy, and parted company on friendly terms.

For a detailed guide to these three stages and other resources on conflict resolution, see Resources at the end of the chapter.

Using Natural Communication

Natural communication provides the skills to express yourself, hear others, have a fruitful conversation. You'll need these skills in conflict resolution and many other situations. All this is closer to gardening than you might think: both need a dynamic approach which accepts conflicts as normal, and seeks to learn and grow through them. You can probably see that the other way, imposing control, suppressing the problems, doesn't work for long. So here are some principles for natural communication:

- *See the situation like a garden:* consider the other person, and your relationship, with a gardener's eye. What is the ground condition, how could it be improved? What do you need to cultivate or prune out? What could be composted?
- *Grow from the roots:* if your connection with this person is tricky, how could you nourish its roots, give it some positive energy for new growth?
- *Observation:* a gardener looks closely at what is, and avoids getting lost in emotional drama or their own needs and mindset. As Stephen Covey says, 'Seek first to understand, then to be understood.'
- *Accept decline and endings:* in Nature, we see decay and death all the time, but we humans find them hard to accept in our lives. Maybe you need to talk about a relationship or project which is in decline, or has reached its end. Recognise this can be hard for everyone involved.
- *Use heart and head:* gardeners are great role models for combining love with skill and intelligence.
- *Make space for pauses:* someone at work in a garden will pause regularly to reflect and let intuition contribute. This can make stickier conversations easier too. Try suggesting a couple of minutes of reflective quiet at the start, or anytime tension is rising.

You'll find more on natural communication techniques in Resources. Here's an overview of the main elements, drawn from a range of leading experts:

- *Clean communication and assertiveness:* simple ways to make your point clearly and acceptably; for example, using 'I' statements, not generalising or blaming
- *Body language:* understanding and using it well; for example, making eye contact
- *Good listening:* ways to ensure that you really hear the other person, and that they feel heard
- *Giving negative feedback:* this is notoriously hard to do well, but there are methods which can help
- *Receiving criticism:* pointers to help you hear and consider critical comments, without blowing up!

Won't Get Fooled Again: Change the Story
Paula's Story: men always put you down

When she was a young child, Paula remembers how her dad was angry and dissatisfied with her mum, on the rare times he was home.

Paula's dad left when she was 6, and her mum became depressed and unsupportive. In adult life, Paula's partners put her down and left her repeatedly, and she had similar bosses at work.

By midlife, Paula had a long history of depression, but eventually realised she was repeating a Story which she could choose to change.

One of my biggest insights in recent years has been the way repeating stories shape our lives. So what do I mean by a Story? Most of us have one or two major repeating, difficult patterns in our life. We may not be aware of them, we may not call them a Story, but they shape our experiences. Most often, a Story begins with a major upset in childhood. Our subconscious mind tries to explain and justify that first upset by repeating the situation. See Paula's Story in the box for an example.

This kind of Story is not logical: it's usually not even something we're aware of. It's a primitive survival tool from early years. If you're still repeating a Story like this, it will be a deeply ingrained habit, and you'll need a sustained effort to shift it. You may know about neural pathways: old habits become physically imprinted within our brain, so they are truly hard to change. But the payback to doing so is that it can transform the way you handle life.

A repeating Story means that you don't see situations as they are, because you're unconsciously shaping them to fit your Story. Changing a major life Story may need professional help from a counsellor or therapist. Most of us have at least one major Story, and some minor ones. For example, look at your beliefs and habits around money, or food, or health. The self-help process below is designed to assist you in seeing and changing your Stories. Try it on a minor one first!

Self-help Process: Changing a Story

Set aside at least 40 minutes for this process, and find a quiet time and place where you won't be interrupted.

Take some long, slow breaths. Make sure you breathe out fully. Let yourself relax.

Now start to remember a few significant experiences around a current difficult situation, or some aspect of your life you've chosen to explore, or for your life as a whole.

If this is distressing, keep breathing deeply, aim to witness the emotions and let them go.

Now start to look or listen for a pattern, a repeating feeling or Story. Give this time, be patient and receptive. If nothing comes up, go back over the scenes again.

What you're aiming to find is a simplistic, sweeping statement that feels horribly powerful to you, and probably makes you tense up. A good sign that you've found it is if it has words like *always, never, can't, no good*.

Be very gentle with yourself, don't blame or judge yourself for carrying this Story for so long. Be grateful you've found the courage to name it and face it now.

The next step is to find an antidote to your Story: a simple, positive statement that you can affirm whenever the negative beliefs come up.

Here are some examples of negative Stories and an affirmation as an antidote to them:

- *Men/women always let me down: I fully deserve love and loyalty*
- *I'm just not good enough: I always do my best and deserve support*
- *People never respect me: I have all the strength and safety I need*

It helps to repeat frequently the affirmations you've chosen. And if something upsets you, use the situation to see what Story it's showing you. Trust that you can change your Story, and choose a happy one.

Easing the Bumps

Minor, everyday challenges and even major ones can have an upside. They're another chance to identify your Story, or to practise changing it. If you've already named your Story, sometimes you'll realise you're repeating it, while it's happening, and you can compost it in the moment. Try taking a few breaths, a loo break, any way to give yourself a bit of space, and see how you can do things differently, in the here and now.

Often our relationships have a Story too: especially with partners, family, close friends and work colleagues. You can use the self-help process above for these situations too. It can also work for groups, such as a work team or community group.

If you can see a Story between you and someone else, what can you do about it? At minimum, get clearer how your behaviour causes the Story to repeat, and try to change it. If you're feeling calm and brave, and there's good rapport between you, try naming the Story to the other person. Present it as simply your impression, ask them what they think. Even if they have a different view, you'll have learned something and deepened your connection.

If you can find agreement, you've got a powerful way to improve the relationship. I recall a stormy period with a girlfriend where we'd regularly pause in mid-argument, and say, 'We're doing it again!' People love stories: it's how we make sense of life. So remember, the aim is to *replace* a negative Story with a positive one. Look for a simple, hopeful statement which lifts your spirits, is easy to remember, and which you can repeat to yourself often. It will raise the prospects of a Story with a happy outcome!

Resources

Here are some ways to explore the topics in this chapter more fully.

Feel the Fear and Do It Anyway, by Susan Jeffers. If you need to do some deep emotional composting, this self-help book could be useful.

Conflict Resolution: there is a detailed version of this three-step process in the Resources section of **https://www.naturalhappiness.net**

Conflicts: A Better Way to Resolve Them, by Edward de Bono. A clear and practical guide to conflict resolution.

Natural communication techniques: you'll find a fuller guide to these in the Resources section of **https://www.naturalhappiness.net**

How to be Assertive in Any Situation, by Sue Hadfield and Gill Hasson. One of the most highly rated books on the topic. It provides a good grounding in communication and assertiveness skills for relationships and other situations.

Non-Violent Communication, by Marshall Rosenberg. A brilliant book: *NVC* is much more widely relevant than the name suggests. There are also training groups and support networks based on *NVC.* See **https://liferesources.org.uk**

Helpguide.org: a good website for basic relationship skills, including topics like emotional intelligence, and understanding anger and conflict resolution. Their Emotional Intelligence Toolkit is also good. See: **https://www.helpguide.org**

Chapter 4

Shaping Uncertainty: The Co-creative Way

Most people are trying to shape their lives amid more uncertainty than they can handle: co-creative skills make this easier. It's about finding solutions *with* other people's needs, *with* apparent obstacles, *with* uncertainty, balancing them with your own needs and hopes. We may wish we could get on top of things and take control, but we're living in turbulent times where co-creative approaches are a better option.

This has been hard for me to learn. I started my career with American marketing giant Procter and Gamble. We were expected to make it happen, drive things forward, crush the obstacles. Even the business world has learned that real life's not like that, as shown by best-selling books like *Thriving on Chaos*.

I moved straight from directing a large business to starting an organic farm. It was a massive shock. An organic farmer's work is like driving a tractor without a steering wheel: he or she can't *make* anything happen. It's a continuous juggle between the realities of the weather, the soil, and what you'd like to achieve. Magdalen Farm was my biggest teacher of co-creative ways.

You probably know the idea of fight or flight: the co-creative approach is a third way: I call it dancing with the problem, or listening for a different view. This chapter starts with stories, to show the idea in practice. Then you'll find a section on principles, a toolkit of techniques, and ways to manifest a vision.

Co-creative Stories

Previous chapters have explored gardening techniques that you can learn from, like composting or crop rotation. Here we shift focus to the way a gardener or farmer relates to their land, and subtle human skills which may help you.

Co-creating in the Garden

My wife Linda and I spend a lot of time tending the 1-acre garden of our home in West Dorset. It's much improved since we moved here in 2010: we lived with frustrations about the garden for a year, so we could observe it in all weathers, and evolve a plan that grew from the place. Early on, Linda's ideas and mine were alarmingly different. It was time in the garden that brought a consensus between the two of us and the land.

Linda and I are in the garden most days: not just to enjoy it, but engaged in an almost continuous, wordless conversation with it. We're observing what's growing, what's struggling, and listening for the message in the situation. Some gardeners talk of listening to the land and their plants: we do this, but it's more of a dialogue, because we're imagining how to react to what we hear, putting out questions and requests for guidance, and seeking feedback on our plans. This is a good example of co-creativity in action. Here are a few specific examples:

Companion planting: instead of poisoning the pests, bring in plants which distract or deter them. We have nasturtiums in our brassica bed, because cabbage white butterflies are attracted to them and leave the vegetables alone. We've planted calendula and basil near our tomatoes because whitefly dislike them and avoid the area.

Transforming an eyesore: when we bought our house, it came with a disused outdoor swimming pool. We felt embarrassed by this eyesore, and started asking for help from what we'd call the wisdom of the garden. At last an idea bubbled up: to create a sunken garden. Instead of removing all that concrete, we had it broken up and covered with topsoil. Going down into this area creates a feeling of secluded space, and it's now full of colour and fragrance.

Sharing the bounty: a co-creative approach means considering the needs of all parties involved. We protect parts of our crop from birds, but leave some for them. Our cherry tree was getting stripped as soon as the fruit started to colour. So we wrapped the lower half in fleece, but left the upper half as a giveaway.

Restraining the thugs: I need to set on record that Linda has more technical gardening expertise than me, and does more of the work in the garden. So here's her take on co-creating: 'I see my role as a kind of crowd control, restraining the thugs and ensuring fair play for the slow growers. The thugs may be quite pretty, like geraniums, but they stifle variety if you don't intervene. Plants put themselves where they want to be — you have to decide whether to go along with it.'

Co-creating on the Farm

When you're cultivating plants or animals, you can't get it 100 per cent right. In one sense, an organic farmer's life is a string of 'failures', and I've always been humbled by their resilience. Clearly, they get comfort from their love of the land, from their successes, and by knowing that natural life is cyclical. Here are a couple of co-creative stories from Magdalen Farm.

Send in the pigs: On one of our farm walks, I stopped at a field that was getting choked with weeds, and asked Peter, our farm manager, 'What are we going to do with this problem?' He replied, 'Send in the pigs,' and explained: 'Sometimes in farming when you have a bit of a mess, the best solution is to make a bigger mess. The pigs will make a mud heap of it, but they'll destroy the weeds and dung it up, then we can start over.'

There are no failures: just revisions: A natural system has no waste, and no failures: if the crop you planned for has problems, you just find another way to use it. A failed crop can be used as animal feed, or composted as a green manure.

Listening to your problems: In conventional farming, weeds will be killed with herbicide. But Peter used to tell me, 'Every weed species has a message for us. If you observe which weeds grow where, they'll show us what remedial action the earth is calling for.'

Principles of Co-creativity

When I teach co-creative approaches, people like the idea, but find it elusive in practice. This section offers some guiding principles:

- Use and explore tensions constructively: for example, between your wishes and the realities. Learn to live with conflicts and use the stress to move you forward.
- Intensify your commitment, i.e. feel fully involved in the situation, and deeply wanting a resolution, even though you can't see it. This usefully increases the creative tension, see more below.
- Harness all the wisdom in the situation: for example, by some form of dialogue with the apparent problem, whether that's a person or a situation. This is explored in the self-help Quickie below, on Befriending your problem.
- Find ways to integrate both analytical, logical skills and your intuition. This is sometimes described as using both sides of the brain. The Diamond Process is one way to do this, explained later in this chapter.
- Give the whole process time: in particular, relaxing, letting go of the issue consciously, so that your subconscious has space to contribute.
- Call in higher guidance in some way, possibly through prayer: this is explored more in Chapter 7.
- Look out for, and write down as soon as you can, brief flashes of intuition, apparently silly ideas that pop into your head, and dreams. They may be how your subconscious responds!
- Try to notice your own limiting beliefs and blind spots which prevent you seeing wider possibilities. This is where changing the Story comes in (see Chapter 3).
- Embrace complexity, include different voices or factors in the situation, and within yourself, even if they seem contradictory.

- Deepen your observation, so you can use subtle and peripheral data to work with a fuller picture: for example, through Tracker Vision, covered later in this chapter.
- Draw on all your faculties, including inspiration, playfulness and naivety.
- Access wider sources of insight: including other people and the natural world.

Using Tension Creatively

Tension and uncertainty often provoke a fight-or-flight response, an urge to find a quick solution or walk away. The co-creative response to a dilemma or a setback is to relax into it and explore it. There are many ways to do this: deep, relaxed breathing is a good one to try, or going for a walk. Review your own needs, feelings, ideas, and those of the person who seems to be blocking you.

Sometimes you need to intensify the tension, not relax into it. The more you *feel* the tension, the stronger the stimulus for your intuition to resolve it. Reality can often feel complex and overwhelming: usually we limit what we take in, but we may miss out on creative insights. Our brain is wired to simplify life by putting new experiences into a category of past ones, which means we can easily believe we're in a negative pattern, a repeating Story. I recommend the Change the Story process in Chapter 3 to explore this.

Real life is full of contradictions. Think about a major new event, like the 2020 pandemic. You probably had conflicting reactions, such as fear and curiosity. And you had to deal with widely differing opinions from others. So much complexity is hard to live with: we often react by putting on blinkers, ignoring a lot of information, or by apathy, giving up on the effort to understand. Learning to relax into the tension will help with this, and there are processes which can help you: for example, the Diamond Process below.

Drawing on Both Sides of the Brain

One way of developing co-creativity is through harnessing the left and right sides of the brain. The talents of the left side include logic, reasoning, the ability to analyse a complex situation. The right side of the brain offers intuition and imagination. While the left brain can dissect a complex situation, break it into smaller parts by analysis, it is the right side that gives us creative vision, a different approach, the fresh combination of parts to move us forward. The Diamond Process below can help you use both sides together.

Try consciously to use both sides. I have a quick analytical mind, so I frequently need to slow myself down. If you're more naturally intuitive, try asking yourself logical questions. One of my favourite ways to use the whole brain is what I call Park and Ride. Start by thinking analytically about a problem, gather facts, questions, puzzles. Then stop fretting: park the problem, do something else, and usually the intuition pops up with an answer.

Linda and I are constantly combining analysis and intuition in our gardening: for example, if a new problem arises like rust on the onions, or peach leaf curl, our first steps are usually logical, gathering facts from garden books or websites. Intuition helps us decide if this is serious enough to intervene, or if the plants can cope with it unaided. And we're also using intuition to look for a 'systemic' solution, like a need for more crop rotation, or a change to our composting methods.

Your Co-creative Toolkit

This section offers some of the favourite processes I've evolved to apply the co-creative approach. Just as you build up new muscles gradually to play a new sport, try these methods on your smaller challenges to start with.

The Diamond Process

The Diamond Process offers a framework for using both sides of the brain. It's relevant for issues of many kinds, including practical, big-picture, or emotional.

The shape of the diamond symbolises the shape of most change processes. There is a starting point: an intention, a question. From this point, the picture widens into growing uncertainty and contradiction. A successful change process finds new insight that gives clarity, bringing us to a finishing point, which in turn will often be the start of another diamond.

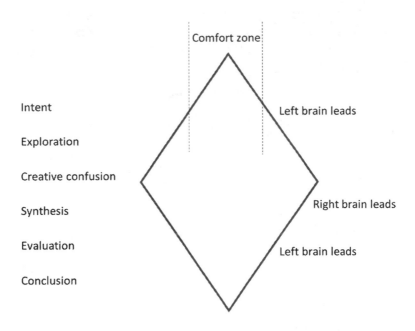

The six stages in the process are as follows.

1. Intent

You plant the seed for this process by stating and affirming your intent. Even if your aim is as vague as 'to understand my confusion', state this explicitly. This calls in and engages your intuition. The same approach is expounded by Timothy

Gallwey in his book *The Inner Game of Tennis:* the logical brain specifies the goal, but never prescribes how to achieve it. It briefs the intuitive mind to find the solution.

2. Exploration

In each phase of the Diamond Process, both sides of the brain may contribute but one takes the lead. Here it is the active, logical, left brain. This is the stage for gathering data, exploring a range of information sources, analysing what's going on, looking for relevant parallels. One aim is to go beyond your comfort zone: the habitual frame of reference and limiting beliefs that we use to reduce the confusions of real life to a manageable level.

3. Creative Confusion

If your exploratory work has been done well, it will naturally propel you into confusion: you'll feel overloaded with contradictory information. The word confusion literally means a flowing together, and the aim in this stage is to relax into the tension and uncertainty: to feel its intensity and to stay with it. Resist the desire to find a solution.

4. Synthesis

This is the phase when you open receptively to the 'aha!' moment, the insight that produces a way forward from the confusion. Like any right-brain process, you can't force it. Sometimes just closing your eyes, breathing peacefully, and waiting enables you to find the synergy. This is a good time to go for a walk, have a bath, sit in the garden: do something enjoyable and stay observant for the answer when it's ready.

5. Evaluation

Here the left brain takes the lead again. From stage 4, you should have a vision of an outcome: you need to check out the practicalities, do the sums, ask the questions, consult others. None of us have 100 per cent infallible intuition, and you may have to return to an earlier phase of the cycle to check things out.

6. Conclusion

Your evaluation may support your new vision, or highlight doubts or risks. Before you go ahead, return to the right brain: sit with your potential decision, see if it inspires and motivates you. This is the stage where we often say: 'I'll sleep on it.' It is sometimes wise to cycle back within this process and repeat some stages. For example, the creative confusion stage may raise more questions to explore. It's also cyclical because the conclusion to one diamond often becomes the starting point for another.

Self-help Quickie: Befriending Your Problem

This exercise might take 20–30 minutes. You'll need a friend or colleague to do it with: don't choose someone directly involved in the situation you're exploring. Both of you should read the instructions below a couple of times, then try to do the process from memory.

Don't spend time briefing your partner about the situation. Trust that their intuition will provide the insights you need. This process can help you understand a problem or obstacle you'd like to resolve. Ask your partner to represent the problem — they don't need to know what it is in any detail. Explain that you're just asking them to follow any impulses about how to move or what to say during the process.

Stand facing each other. Notice how you feel as you look at each other. Then come closer, and bring your forearms into contact — just hold each other's elbows, with eyes shut.

For a few minutes, stand like this silently, with eyes closed. You imagine you're meeting your problem in person. Your partner notices how they feel about you, and reports this at the end: it may help you understand your problem better.

When you feel ready, tell your partner that you can both make small movements. Keep your eyes closed, and your forearms in contact. Notice if one of you is more pushy or more passive. Observe any feelings that come up.

Tracker Vision and Fox Walk

Some of our programmes at Hazel Hill Wood teach wilderness skills, like tracking and fire-making, which humans have used for thousands of years to survive in the wild. In many ways, our brains and bodies are still geared up for the Stone Age, and that's why these primitive skills can offset some of the confusion of twenty-first century screen world

I'm using the term tracker vision to cover a range of skills which can help us to slow down and deepen our observation in any situation. Gardeners and organic farmers do this too, but it's the wilderness version I'd like to explore. In primitive times, the ability to track animals, to hunt them or avoid them, was basic to survival, so evolution has created humans who are naturally good at this!

These days, many of us spend hours each day in a deluge of data from our smartphone or computer: using our left brains at great speed, but ignoring our other talents. The first aim with tracker vision is to slow right down, connect with all our senses and both sides of our brain. If you're struggling with a thorny problem in any part of your life, I suggest you get outdoors and connect with tracker vision, so that all your faculties can help you find a solution. Ideally do this in the wild woods, but a secluded, overgrown garden or park could do!

Here are the basic elements of tracker vision:

- Use the Fox Walk described below, so that you slow right down, and start to open your senses.
- Take time to connect with all your senses: the sounds of the birds, the smells of outdoors, the taste and touch of Nature.
- If you have a question you need help with, name it, then park it in your subconscious, and take it for a walk.
- Continue to use the Fox Walk, and soften your vision to take in areas to your side. Try to 'see' a 180-degree range, but in a receptive, observant way.
- You may want to find a 'sit spot', a tree or clearing, and stay in this wide-angle, observant state. Wait for insights to arise, as a fisherman waits.

The Fox Walk

Fox-walking steps are best done in bare feet (or thin-soled shoes), using the bones, muscles and sensitivity of your feet to their full potential.

Lift up one leg until your thigh is parallel to the ground. Then let the foot come down softly to the ground so the ball, not the heel, touches first. The bones and tendons will stretch slowly to take your weight, minimising the shockwaves going through body and earth. Spread your weight along the outer edge of your foot to the heel, and when your body weight is all on this foot, slowly lift up the other foot, as a heron does, from the top of the ankle, to repeat the process again with the other leg. As you move, especially if there are other people, obstacles or trees and undergrowth around, you will be developing spatial awareness and exerting great body control. Your awareness spreads as you feel your way through your feet, becoming aware, with the edge of your vision, of suitable places for your feet to fall, and negotiating branches with slow, whole-body movement.

Once, as I was fox-walking along a hedgerow at the edge of a scrubby field, a fox got up from where it had been dozing. It stretched and sloped off, in no particular rush at all, under a low holly branch. I had not really disturbed it, just got too close for its comfort. If I had been wandering along at a usual walking pace, the fox would have been long gone before I reached its resting place. As we slow down to nature speed and allow our whole selves to be present, we can refocus on the world outside to develop peripheral awareness and allow our brainwaves to change to a more relaxed and natural pattern.

When fox-walking I certainly find a great deal of peacefulness and inner stillness. Sometimes I get ideas, have insights and inspiration, because I am moving slowly and quietly enough to notice them; the wild ideas on the inside, as well as the wildlife on the outside. Fox-walking is one of the ultimate walking meditations, being totally present and aware, moving very slowly and blending into the landscape. You too will see more wildlife and feel enlivened if you give it a go.

Reprinted with permission from 'I Love My World' by Chris Holland, published by Wholeland Press.

Play, Dance and Dream with Your Problems

All kinds of creativity can help in your co-creative toolkit. Here are a few I can recommend:

- *Fun:* Use play and humour to get new insights. Where's the funny side in the situation? How would *Spitting Image* depict it?
- *Reality shift:* If your problem is someone you find difficult and scary, change perspective. Imagine waltzing with them and having a cosy chat. Or picture them with a long, warty nose; they won't seem so scary.
- *Reverse thrust:* Ask yourself the question, and even brainstorm, how to achieve the *opposite* of the intended outcome. For example, 'how could I make this hospital as unwelcoming to patients as possible?' Reversing the ideas generated should yield some fresh approaches to the desired goal.
- *Role playing:* This can free you from preconceived positions, and bring in new points of view. For example, imagine the positions of various people involved with a project, and then actually play each role in turn, imagining what constructive solutions each of them would suggest. You can use this not only for various people around you, but also to represent different aspects of yourself: for example, your ambitious aspect, your lazy aspect, your inner critic, your creative self, and so on. Moving to a different seat for each role can help you connect with them.
- *Dream:* Ask for a dream to guide you. When you go to bed, ask out loud for help, name your questions, put paper and pen by the bed to show you mean it. If you wake with a dream in the night, write it down, and try to make sense in the morning.
- *Call for help:* Meditate and call for guidance. Call in help from anyone you trust: a friend, a mentor, a saint. Ask for insights that serve everyone involved, not just your own needs, and leave plenty of time for the answer to come.

How Nature Helps Co-creativity

Nature contact is a crucial antidote to screen time, which sucks up our attention and limits our creativity. *Your Brain on Nature* is a book by two doctors at Harvard Medical School which gathers extensive research evidence on the problems of screen world, and how Nature can offset them. Directed Attention Fatigue describes the mental drain and stress which arise from a sustained effort of giving our attention to a task or situation. It's aggravated when your attention is frequently distracted by new information from text messages, emails and so on.

If you suspected that screen world is addictive, this book confirms it: 'We are wired to crave information — big time . . . The brain uses dopamine to reward information seeking.' However, Nature contact is an effective antidote. Research shows that Nature experiences have 'intrinsic fascination', hence they are a counterbalance to many modern stresses. Time in Nature actually induces positive feelings, which can outweigh stress and anxiety, and stimulate our creativity.

You may recall from the Tree Test in Chapter 1 that when a tree is under stress, it deepens its roots. We humans need to do the same, and spending more time with Nature is part of this. So too are stronger links with family, friends and community, and with faith and belief.

Weaving Multiple Viewpoints

My favourite poet, T.S. Eliot, wrote that 'humankind cannot bear much reality'. A common way to cope with complexity is to simplify, to polarise it into two apparently opposed positions. Even my co-creative material risks suggesting that you need to resolve tension between just two positions: your wishes and the situation you face. However, we ourselves may have various, conflicting opinions and feelings. The situation, or the other people, may well be complex too. Plus, there's fake news, and social media trying to manipulate us for profit.

Consider your experience of gardens: they are dynamic, living ecosystems which need to be considered from a variety of viewpoints. And a gardener needs to engage a range of energies (physical, emotional, mental, inspirational) and skills to handle this complexity: such as observation, patience and intuition.

Another way that the garden metaphor can help us here is with the idea of listening for insights from non-human sources. Tuning in to hear the 'voice' of your garden, of a tree, of a vegetable bed, is important to many gardeners. I use this method with all my work: listening to insights from the 'voice' of a work team, a project, a problem.

The third source I find helpful is what could be summed up as higher guidance. This can take many forms, depending on your preferences and beliefs. You could simply call on your higher self, your deepest intuition, to give you a perspective. Or you could pray for insight. My belief is that there are subtle, intangible sources of wisdom we can connect with, and I'll explore this further in Chapter 7.

The Circle of Voices process is one that I have evolved, drawing on these three sources. You should be able to adapt this to a range of situations, and to using it with other people if they are up for it. You could see this method as a version of the Diamond Process described earlier in the chapter. What's different here are structured ways of bringing in various aspects of a situation, hopefully the hidden as well as the obvious. It can help you to recognise contradictions in your own views, to understand other viewpoints better and to get bigger perspectives; for example, from the vision of the project itself. You'll find the Circle of Voices process in the Appendix.

Manifestation

I'm using this word to mean the ability to bring a vision or idea to fruition. My success at achieving this with several ambitious projects continues to surprise me. There's no simple formula to share, but this is my best attempt to explain what I do. It's important to add that I've also launched some initiatives which have gone nowhere, despite all my best efforts! This description draws mainly on big projects that I've initiated, but I use a version of this for small projects, like creating a weekend retreat, also for relationships, and to see how I can best contribute to projects where I'm not the leader.

Nature has a large but often invisible influence in manifestation as I've experienced it. Much of my learning about this topic, and co-creativity generally, came from spending time at the Findhorn Foundation, an ecovillage and spiritual community in Scotland. Starting from one rented caravan, what they have manifested is amazing, and dialogue with Nature played a vital role. It's an inspiring story, and you'll find books about it in Resources.

Listen for guidance and follow it: you can guess from this book that I spend a fair bit of time in a receptive state, usually in Nature, where insights can reach me most easily. I need to do this by deliberate choice, because by temperament I'm a self-driving person who likes to make things happen. The big project ideas usually arise when I'm not looking for them. My approach is simply to live with these ideas for weeks or longer, and see if they persist. Often they seem alarmingly ambitious, as well as exciting, and one of my responses is a prayer to say, 'If you really want me to take this on, you need to show me the people and resources to do it with.'

One of my tests of whether to act on a big idea is to watch for synchronicities: if help shows up, often from unexpected sources, I take it as a sign to keep going. I believe that a real willingness to act on the guidance you receive is vital if you want to continue receiving like this.

Carry the vision, but reshape the form: when a big idea shows up, it's usually a broad vision, and part of my role is to evolve the form it takes. For example, Magdalen Farm is a 130-acre farm with residential facilities and numerous sub-projects. It started as a powerful but vague image, like a Turner watercolour sunrise. I understood this as a catalytic project involving Nature contact for young people: it took several months of exploring real-life possibilities and listening for more guidance before it evolved into the form we manifested.

This reshaping is a classic co-creative process. You could call my role the vision holder: this involves carrying the dream, trying to discern its essence and explore the form it is calling for. Keeping the sense that you're in service to some bigger concept which is coming through you is vital. If your ego or will tries to take charge, you'll lose the original inspiration. As a vision holder, you also need to stay open to a sense that the vision itself needs to be reshaped, or even that you should drop it completely. Sometimes I've carried an inspiring idea around for a few weeks, and then felt I was just meant to lay it to rest: a bit like an interesting house guest who passes briefly through your life.

Keep the vision animated: in order to reach fulfilment, a vision needs its vitality and magnetism maintained. A vision community can help (see more on this below) but if a vision has come through you, you need to keep animating it. One of the main ways I do this is in daily meditation: spending some time connecting with the vision, and bringing it to life: for example, imagining its fulfilled form as vividly as I can. For a workshop group, I help to manifest participants by picturing the group in a session, with the number of people I'm aiming for, and feeling the atmosphere of the workshop.

Tim Smit's book *Eden* is a gripping account of how he manifested a huge, pioneering idea against all the odds. He writes passionately about the Tinkerbell Effect: in *Peter Pan*, Tinkerbell and all the fairies can only live if children believe in them. You have to keep affirming your faith in the (apparently) impossible dream, and the more people do this, the better.

Gather a vision community: this is another idea I picked up at Findhorn. You need one or a few vision holders, and around them it's desirable to form a vision community. This is a group of people who help to animate the vision, who may bring in some of the insights or contacts it needs, and who support the vision at crunch times. For example, if there's a major decision to take, or a crisis meeting, ask the members of the vision community to tune in, pray, visualise an outcome that serves the highest good of the situation. They could act as an occasional advisory group, or could just focus on 'holding the vision'.

Be alert for subtle intuitions: manifesting something significant probably requires you to defy logic, and go beyond what looks possible: where will you get the insights to do this? I've found it's essential to keep listening for whispers, for intuitions which may look silly at first. My rule of thumb is that when an idea pops up for the third time, I take it seriously, however much my logic dismisses it.

Keep service to your clients as a guiding focus: in a challenging situation, our ego, or our negative Story, can dominate our reactions, and that's true for other people involved too. From the outset, maintain a strong sense of who you are trying to serve, and how: this should keep you anchored in real life, and also provides a point of reference when strong personalities start to disagree. Over the years, I've realised that many conflicts apparently about the facts really arose from strong personalities needing to be heard, wanting an impact. Having a higher purpose can offset this: and ensuring people feel their views are witnessed helps too!

Learn and grow through setbacks: annealing is a process of strengthening metal by heating and cooling it. Setbacks can have a similar function for human activities. If you're a vision holder or leader, try to accept challenges as a way of testing the project and showing where it needs strengthening.

This is probably hardest if the setback is an attack on your leadership, or even on your vision. Biting criticism of leaders is common in our times, and I still find it very upsetting. The approaches in Chapter 3 have helped: composting the emotions, and giving some time to assess where my limitations are the issue, and where I need to change. This is also where a vision community can give you both perspectives and support.

Maintain yourself as a clear channel: my guess is that someone who's heavily into drink, drugs or other distractions will struggle to sustain a vision or hear the subtle messages. Look after your own wellbeing, keep exercising to burn off stress, and get whatever emotional support you need.

Resources

Drawing on the Right Side of the Brain, by Betty Edwards, published by Souvenir Press. This delightful book gives you the gist of the original research about the two sides of the brain, and the drawing exercises are a good way to stimulate your general creativity.

I Love My World, by Chris Holland, published by Wholeland Press: Chris is a leading UK teacher of wilderness skills and Nature awareness. The book is a great collection of outdoor learning activities, fun for adults as well as kids, including the Fox Walk.

Cultural Emergence by Looby McNamara: this book by a leading permaculture teacher offers some great systemic approaches and processes for applied co-creativity.

Your Brain on Nature, by Alan Logan and Eva Selhub. Subtitled The Science of Nature's Influence on your Health, Happiness and Vitality. A well-researched, persuasive explanation of what screen world is doing to us and how Nature is the best antidote.

Circle of Voices: you'll find a briefing on the process and how to use it in the Appendix at the end of this book.

The Findhorn Garden: this book was written by several members of the Findhorn Community. Aptly subtitled Pioneering a New Vision of Humanity and Nature in Cooperation, it will show you why Findhorn has been such a major inspiration for me.

In Perfect Timing: this autobiography by Peter Caddy, one of the co-founders of Findhorn, is a detailed exposition of how he learned and applied manifestation principles.

Chapter 5

Cultivating Community

The future outlook seems so uncertain and confusing that it's hard to know how to prepare for it. However, almost everyone agrees that raising resilience in communities will help. As Rob Hopkins, founder of the Transition movement, says: 'If we wait for governments, it will be too late. If we act as individuals, it will be too little. But if we act as communities, it might just be enough, and it might just be in time.'

There's a lot we humans can learn from Nature about fruitful communities, and we'll explore this in the first section of the chapter. The second section considers how to raise resilience in communities, with examples from a range of projects. The third helps you explore your relationship with different kinds of communities. The final section offers a community-building toolkit.

In essence, a community is any group of people with a shared purpose. The main focus in this chapter is neighbourhoods, local communities, as they have a big role in our future resilience. You are probably part of several communities, such as family, work or sports teams, faith or environmental groups.

Community in Nature

Ecosystems depend on many aspects of community to thrive and withstand setbacks. To bring these ideas to life, get onto the land, or at least imagine doing so. In my workshops, I sometimes invite people to picture their life as a whole, or their position in a community, as an ecosystem and then map it. To do this, imagine a community group or some other situation as a garden, a farm, or a forest, and draw a picture in which elements of a natural system represent parts of it. For example, a vegetable garden could represent the task functions of the group, an orchard the longer-term work, a neglected woodland glade could signify the vision that you don't connect with enough. By creating a drawing, you make it easier to translate ecosystem features to meet your needs, such as wild margins or companion planting.

Another approach to using the Gardener's Way with communities is to imagine yourself as a gardener, and the group as the garden. Even if you're not the leader, this can be helpful. It enables me to accept people's quirks and independent thinking in the same way that I recognise that each plant or tree has a will of its own. And when I think of cultivating a group, my approach becomes more patient and co-creative.

Community on the Farm

Traditionally, most British agriculture was based on smallish mixed farms, with a range of enterprises: vegetables, arable crops and livestock — maybe 20 milking cows, a few pigs, chickens and so on. These days, most British agriculture is industrial scale, dependent on a single crop or type of livestock. I share the view that smaller mixed farms can provide a better balance of fair productivity, high sustainability and good resilience. Some of these farms have had remarkable results in carbon sequestration too.

Here are some of the community approaches we humans can learn from:

Supportive enterprises: On a mixed farm, the activities support each other. Arable crops provide food and bedding for livestock, and animals provide manure to fertilise the fields. Crop rotation renews the land without chemicals. And diversity adds resilience: if one enterprise fails, others should still support you. For human communities, this highlights the value of diverse skills and mutual support.

Wild margins: This is one of my favourite principles in organic systems. To qualify for organic certification, a farm must leave some field corners and edge land wild, uncultivated. These margins are a haven for wildflowers, plants, birds, insects. Diversity of wildlife and plants has many benefits for humans; for example, if a new pest or disease affects your plants, you can hope that its antidote is hanging out in the wild margins.

How does this work for communities? I've seen many groups who find it hard to include and tolerate divergent and challenging views. The problem is aggravated because 'wild margin' people often feel isolated, angry, and may lack the communication skills to make their points diplomatically. When a group feels threatened and criticised, it's tempting to turn against minority members, to scapegoat or exclude them.

One benefit of the wild margins analogy is to show the potential insights in divergent views. If the majority of a group can learn patience and skills to hear the essence under challenging language, they will access more wisdom and solutions. Nelson Mandela, in solitary confinement for many years on Robben Island, seemed an unlikely person to resolve apartheid in South Africa, but mainstream society's crises are often solved from an unlikely and marginal source.

Community-supported agriculture: for many organic market gardens and farms, there's a fuzzy boundary between who's staff and who's customers. Community-supported agriculture (CSA) means that customers commit to buy a share of whatever produce there is, for a weekly subscription, and they also put in some time as volunteers to help with production, harvesting and packing. This means that producers have assured income even if harvests are poor, and they can keep their prices affordable. It's a great role model for a more fluid, collaborative approach which a lot of human communities will need in future.

Community in the Forest

Ever since my connection with Hazel Hill Wood began in 1987, I experience the wood as a community in many ways: read Peter Wohlleben's book *The Hidden Life of Trees,* which provides ample research evidence. Here are some qualities we can learn from.

The fellowship of trees: Wohlleben's book quotes research to show that trees have some ability to sense, respond and communicate so they form living communities. A solo tree can be vulnerable to wind, pests and other threats. Trees use their collective strength: for example, to share nutrients, to warn each other of threats, to absorb and reduce high wind. Societies like Britain over-focus on individuals and fail to teach us the skills for collective living. We need role models, and the woods and forests provide one.

Symbiosis: This term describes mutual support between organisms. Every element of the ecosystem contributes: insects, birds, flowers, trees, and so on. They can provide protection, food, reproduction and more. For example, birds are attracted to a plant with bright berries: they eat them, and scatter the seeds across the forest to expand the plant's presence. We humans often want to see a return when we give something. The insight from symbiosis is that if we all give what we can, without expecting a direct payback, all of our needs are more likely to be met.

Community in the Garden

Especially if you're a gardener, you'll probably see that many of the ideas above apply in gardens too. Let's explore a few more.

Crop rotation: this is an important method for vegetable growers, and for arable farmers. One benefit is *soil health*: by growing different crops each year on a given piece of soil, you reduce the risk of pests and plant diseases. The second is *renewal rotation*: after farmers grow a crop like wheat which demands a lot of nutrients, they renew fertility in the land by growing a crop which has limited income value, but fixes nitrogen from the air into the soil, such as clover.

Both aspects of crop rotation are useful for human communities. Groups who repeat the same activities get stale, and sometimes need to initiate more change deliberately. The idea of following a demanding task by something light or playful is one I use all the time for myself and in groups.

Raising diversity: this helps the resilience of any system. More variety in the crops you grow means that if one or two fail, you have others. In our garden, we plant a couple of different varieties of each crop, such as tomatoes or apple trees. Often a pest or disease only affects one variety. In groups of people, similar approaches or skills may make things flow easily, but you might lack what you need for an unfamiliar challenge. As with wild margins, it's worth making an effort to include people who bring divergent methods and capabilities.

How Nature Brings People Together

There's a growing movement to create community gardens, many of them in neighbourhoods with social and economic hardship. Often these are market gardens, providing healthy, affordable food. They are also havens of peace in urban jungles, lovingly cared for and decorated. These gardens have proved a great way to bring isolated individuals and fragmented neighbourhoods together. If you have a couple of experienced gardeners, everyone else can learn from them. They enable social connections between old and young, and for people with mental or physical health issues. It's a touching example of the benefits of communities that include both Nature and people.

Most of the workshop groups I run are at venues like Hazel Hill Wood, where we can spend a lot of time outdoors, connecting with Nature, not just with each other. People often say they feel a different sense of community, where the humans are in it with all other forms of life. And this leads to new insights, vitality and creativity. So if you want to deepen the community qualities in a group you're involved with, get outdoors!

In my Nature Resilience Immersions for doctors, we faced the issue of how to bring them present, as they arrived rigid with stress, and only functioning on the mental plane. The solution we found was conservation activity. I explained that we wanted to focus them away from sick humans, onto a healthy ecosystem. They loved having an easy physical task with clear results, where they could socialise with each other. Not only did they relax and become present, they also opened from a purely individual focus to a cooperative one. So active gardening is a great way to help a group become a community.

Communities for Resilience

In this second main section, we'll consider how local communities can raise resilience. Having talked with many people about their fears for the future, there seems to be a shared nightmare scenario in which society's norms are swept aside, and people are looting shops to get food. I share these fears, they're one motive behind the community resilience projects I've initiated. However, violent, selfish behaviour is rare in disaster situations: superhuman acts of care for others are much more common. For reassuring evidence on this (for example, after Hurricane Katrina in New Orleans), see the book by Servigne and Stevens in Resources.

Much of this section describes positive projects to grow resilience and mutual support in local communities. Some of these I helped set up, through Seeding our Future, a non-profit project for resilient responses to climate change: see more in Resources.

Since Neanderthal times, the normal human reactions to a shock are fight, flight or freeze. None of these will help us in the future we're facing: this is why resilience is crucial, and some of this must come from groups. So what kind of situations do communities need to prepare for? Here are a few examples:

- Imagine a disaster of your choice, such as flood, wildfire, major food shortages. Emergency services may be overwhelmed: communities will need to organise responses, in particular for those who are elderly or less mobile.
- Some of the ways we can prepare for climate impacts need collective action, for example to set up a local green energy grid or to persuade the local authority to release more land for allotments, or to campaign for action by national government.
- Mental health issues are spreading: local connections and support are one antidote.
- The safety net of public services (such as health care and social workers) could be swamped by demand, and most people can't pay for private providers. It's likely that voluntary services organised within local communities will need to fill these gaps.

Future Conversations

In 2019, Seeding our Future ran successful pilot programmes in disadvantaged communities in Clydeside, Nottingham and Brixton. Each involved eight facilitated workshops, for 10–18 people, at weekly or fortnightly intervals. The aim was to build community resilience skills, especially in response to climate change. Our team created a programme based on our guesses about how to do this, and those ideas largely worked out.

We guessed that the first stages needed to be foundational: group agreements and processes to create trust and a safe space, plus some basic skills in voicing opinions, hearing others and handling conflicts. This all proved valuable: we had to help some individuals through heated rows, about Brexit and more. The third session was held outdoors, using parts of the natural happiness model. The fourth was the most emotionally intense, where we guided the groups through the Deep Ecology process described in Chapter 6. By enabling people to feel their grief, fear and other difficult emotions about the climate crisis, we enabled them to move into active responses.

Next came a session called At Home with the Planet, with briefing on climate change and related issues, helping people identify likely impacts on their neighbourhood. We followed this with two sessions on Community Matters: building skills in group activism and enabling participants to identify and plan for an issue they wanted to act on. The feedback from participants in Future Conversations was excellent, and these programmes highlighted the need to raise the level of community skills for most people.

Strengthening Food Security in Bridport

Since late 2018, I have been involved with Jem Bendell's Deep Adaptation approach to the climate crisis. I share his view that food security is likely to be one of the biggest climate impacts in Britain during the 2020s. Bridport is a market town in Dorset. For this pilot project, which Seeding our Future began in 2019, it has been essential to start patiently, building up collaborative relationships, working with and through other organisations. Most communities have seen a lot of well-intentioned but naive initiatives that burst onto the scene, try for radical change in a few months, and burn out.

This area already has quite a number of organic farms and veg producers plus home growers. Why do we need anything more? Here's our assessment:

- Increasing droughts around the Mediterranean mean that our main suppliers of fruit and veg are at risk
- Jem and others expect a global Multi Breadbasket failure within the next decade, i.e. one or more of the world staple crops like wheat, rice, soya has crop failures in the same year in the handful of countries that produce most of it
- Even in Bridport, most people buy most of their food from supermarkets, who don't procure locally

One way we've developed our project is through meetings open to anyone in the local community: initially in person, then online when Covid happened. These have brought in new ideas and offers of help, such as access to grant funding. You have to accept that most community initiatives are time consuming. Along with the big open meetings, we've had a lot of email conversations. A great idea that emerged from this is Ambassador Allotments: several local allotment holders agreed to try climate-adaptive cultivation methods and crops, and host open afternoons where other home growers could learn from them.

We've had to be patient, to listen very attentively to other voices in this community, and keep reshaping the project to find the best fit, in classic co-creative mode. Working in partnership with a couple of long-established networks in Bridport has given us credibility and helped us get rooted in the local community. Having a Town Council who understand climate issues and food security has also been invaluable.

Another ingredient that has advanced our work is research. We commissioned a major report showing how producers and consumers in South West England can adapt to future climate conditions, through changes in cultivation methods, crops and diet. Our project has already produced some tangible outcomes and hopefully there will be plenty more to come: see Resources for our website. The biggest challenge we face is a systemic one: most people have difficulty changing habits or investing effort to prepare for a problem before it hits them.

More Initiatives to Learn From

Here are brief details of other projects which may be relevant for your situation.

Role models from Scotland: there seems to be more scope for initiative North of the border. See Resources for my favourite book about Scottish community projects, *The New Road*. It's full of positive, practical case studies.

Woodland immersions for doctors: this is another Seeding our Future initiative. Doctors, both in hospitals and GP groups, are a work community under huge stress. At Hazel Hill Wood, we've run several successful resilience programmes for doctors, using parts of the Natural Happiness model plus inputs on the neurophysiology of stress. See Resources for more info.

Cohousing: a brilliantly simple idea — combine self-contained homes with shared facilities, such as a hall for shared meals and socials, a market garden, guest bedrooms. It's sustainable, affordable and companionable. Having helped set up two cohousing communities, I can tell you that in the UK property system, it's often slow and hard to do; however, the idea can be adapted to existing neighbourhoods or groups of low-impact dwellings such as Tiny Homes. Many cohousing projects use a method of decision-making called sociocracy, which you may find useful. See more on this whole topic in Resources.

Facing the 2020s: this is the first community resilience project I started back in 2011. I worked with consultants to understand success stories and future needs in this area. One of the mysteries we explored is why the excellent pilot projects in many aspects of local resilience have not been widely reproduced. A summary of insights is in the Appendix.

You and Your Communities

If you define community quite widely, you are probably part of several. This section can help you assess the groups you're in, and how they fit your needs. I've listed seven kinds of community: review how many of these you're involved in.

1. **Family and friends:** if you think about the benefits of community, you'll hopefully feel you get some of these from family and friends. As the pressures of life grow, bust-ups with people close to us seem to happen more often: one upside of seeing family and friends like this is to use community skills to prevent or heal such conflicts.

2. **Local neighbourhood:** some local neighbourhoods are close-knit communities, others hardly at all. I recall a friend who lived for several years in a street in North London where no one spoke to one another. She rented a hall and invited everyone to a party: over half the residents came, and suddenly it became a community who looked out for each other, loaned stuff, enjoyed each other's company. These days, it's hard to foresee what problems or blessings might affect your neighbourhood, but you'll all be more resilient if you have a stronger sense of community.

3. **Shared interests:** this might include sports clubs, gardening, yoga. Such groups are a kind of community, because you have regular social contact, a sense of fellowship, and some scope for mutual support.

4. **Shared values:** a group with shared values is likely to have deeper trust and insights, and more willingness to help each other in hard times. Examples of shared values

would be a sustainability group like Transition Towns, a Buddhist meditation group, or a cancer support group.

5. **Work organisations:** I admit that many work teams don't have community qualities, but the best teams I've seen did have. This is more likely in a values-based organisation like a social enterprise or charity. Consider if community qualities exist in any work teams you're involved with, and how you'd like to help cultivate them.

6. **Vision community:** this means a group of people drawn together by a shared vision which they want to sustain or bring to fruition. So if you have a big goal, or are supporting someone else with one, this can really help it happen.

7. **Intentional community:** this describes communities with a formal organisation structure, which require people to commit to a code of values, and where people are living together. Intentional communities may be loose-knit, like an ecovillage, or intense, like a commune or a monastery. They're a very useful source of wisdom for informal communities of all kinds; see more in Resources.

You may feel connections with several different scales of neighbourhood: for example, immediate neighbours, those in nearby streets, and the larger settlement you're part of — town, city, village.

Investing time in reviewing and strengthening your community connections can have many benefits. It should raise your resilience for a variety of challenges, and it can meet other needs, such as fellowship, or access to expertise and resources. And it can give you more fulfilment, by providing channels for you to use your talents to help others.

If you'd like to explore this more deeply, see Community Mapping in Resources. On my website you will find a process with worksheet formats to help you identify what you need from communities, and what you can contribute. You can also map how far the communities you're involved with fulfil this, and highlight where you may want to make changes.

Your Community-building Toolkit

Have you ever been in groups that were going nowhere? Perhaps stuck in bickering, blame or fantasy. Where everyone wanted to talk and nobody wanted to listen? There's a vast array of skills, processes, experience which can help communities and other groups be effective and fun. This section offers a selection of these.

Some Essential Tools

Communication skills: these are a foundation for any effective group. The ability to express yourself and hear others, especially for feelings, is vital. Look at the Natural Communication section in Chapter 3 for techniques and further resources.

Facilitation: many groups need more skills and perspective to move forward. Facilitation means enabling: it's a set of skills to support a group to reach an outcome. The facilitator could be a member of the group, or someone independent. See Resources for more.

Ground rules: these could also be called group agreements. Getting group acceptance for ground rules at the start of a gathering can help everyone feel safe and feel heard. Here are some examples:

- Confidentiality: what's said here stays here
- Everyone should have a chance to speak before anyone speaks a second time
- We agree to each speak for ourselves using 'I' statements, rather than speaking for the group

Group Dynamics: over the years, I've realised that what a group discussion is *really* about may not be the apparent topic at all.

People repeat their own dramas in groups, and use them to meet emotional needs, usually covertly. Structure, ground rules, good facilitation can all mitigate the problem, but even better is understanding a bit about group dynamics: see more in Resources.

Conflict Handling: oddly, if you have conflict coming up in your community or other group, you could see this as a sign of progress. It means people feel safe enough to voice disagreements — or are so concerned about the topic that they can't hold back! See Chapter 3 for more on conflict resolution.

Including Fun and Imagination

One reason why Rob Hopkins started the Transition movement was that he found some of the other sustainability networks overly heavy and serious. His book *From What Is to What If* is a great reminder that we need more fellowship, fun and creativity if we want wider involvement and positive change around the climate crisis and other issues.

In our troubled times, it's easy for us to lapse into brain mush, helpless overwhelm, individually and collectively. We have to *choose* play and creativity, and groups can help us to do this, if we can create 'spaces of safety and hope'. Rob cites many projects where giving people an experience of a positive future, enabling them to shape a hopeful story, was a catalyst for actual change. For example, Transition Town Tooting turned an unloved roundabout into a thriving village green for a weekend. The roads were officially closed, turf was laid, bands paraded, kids played games, and the whole neighbourhood saw what was possible.

How Structure Helps

Just as rambling roses and runner beans need a framework to grow on, communities need some structure or they'll sprout into a mess. Clearly some groups need to be more formal than others. But although you may not think of structure with family and friends, you'll have norms and rituals which come to the same thing, like taking it in turns to buy the first round! Informal communities, like a friendship group or a neighbourhood, may be resistant to any talk about skills or structure, and you may need to slide ideas in subtly. Here are some ideas to show how structure can be helpful:

- If meetings are chaotic, suggest two simple guidelines: first, no interruptions, hear each other out; second, everyone must speak once before anyone speaks again.
- Leadership is a good way to bring structure to chaos. Rotating the leadership involves people, and reduces grumbles over hierarchy.
- If you're in a community where conflicts are frequent, you could suggest a simple process, e.g. if two people can't resolve an issue, they both ask another group member to support them in a mediation meeting.
- Whilst structure may sound serious, there are ways of making it fun. I was in a men's group where we designated a 'fireman' for every session, whose role was to hose down (metaphorically!) anyone who got too heated.

Cultivation as a Leadership Art

It was probably a community leader who coined that phrase about herding cats. This is rarely leadership by giving instructions: it's a co-creative process, so the skills in Chapter 4 are relevant here. Cultivating a garden is a good model for leading a community group. You know you're not in control, you know that constant observation and review are needed. You have to choose which issues to tackle and push on, and let go of many. Patience, tolerance, inclusiveness are useful: but you must also know when to take a stand, when to assert values and principles that are under attack. And groups and projects go through the cycle of the four seasons, just as gardens do.

In cultivating a garden, observation of detail really matters, and this is true for communities. Just as you look out for the earliest signs of a plant that's struggling, do the same for people. If you notice and respond promptly, you can avoid widespread unease later. Here's a quote from an American intentional community pioneer, Larry Kaplowitz: 'We've learned that it's the little things — the minor hurts, the petty judgements about each other that undermine and limit the degree of wellbeing in our relationships.'

There's a whole school of thought called Servant Leadership, which urges leaders to see themselves as serving their group and their project. Many gardeners have the humility to see themselves as in service to their garden, and this outlook is a good way to avoid arrogance and egotism. It also suggests that there's always more to learn. In Nature, we accept the cycle of growth and decay, we know that some crops fail. This is a good antidote to our unrealistic ideal of human leaders always succeeding!

Learning from Intentional Communities

People who've known me a long time tell me I've matured and become easier to relate to in recent years. I give much of the credit to my involvement with intentional communities, especially the Findhorn Foundation, a spiritual community and ecovillage in north-east Scotland. Findhorn gave me the inspiration to start the Threshold Centre, the small intentional community and cohousing group in Dorset where I lived for 5 years.

Intentional communities involve people living and working together, trying to fulfil their values: so they're an intense form of group, and they have produced expertise which is relevant for communities and groups of all kinds. They mostly have a vision of community which brings people, Nature and higher purpose together, and we can learn a lot from this. The best distillation of wisdom from this sector that I've found is an American book,

Creating A Life Together (see Resources for details). Here are some insights from this book and my own experiences:

- One section of the book is headed 'The roots of conflict: emotionally charged needs'. This is a crucial insight: what's *under* apparently practical or technical issues is usually emotional. The sooner you see this, and seek to understand and defuse the emotional charge, the easier life will be.
- When I'm facilitating a meeting in any group, I start with a check-in: a short round where everyone can say how they're feeling. Otherwise people act out their difficult emotions until they're so disruptive they have to be noticed.
- Community groups tend to attract sociable people, idealists, and also difficult and needy people who hope the group will make things right like a fantasy parent. If you're in a group which can choose its members, realise there may be times when you have to draw lines and say no to people. It's a very uncomfortable thing for a group to do, but the alternative could be chaos and paralysis. If you have a selection process, make it transparent and fair; for example, a try-out period for all potential members, and review by a sub-group, not one individual.
- Here are two ways to help a group get past its personality differences: one is for everyone to voice their enthusiasm for the highest aims and vision of the group; the other is to get people alarmed about external threats and the consequence of failure.
- The idea of 'structural conflict' can be useful: this means weaknesses of structure in a group, like ambiguous goals or unclear norms and agreements, which make conflict inevitable.

- If you are choosing a group (e.g. for a vision community), include people with emotional maturity, don't look only for technical or professional skills.

Community and Work Organisations

Does the idea of community qualities in work organisations sound far-fetched to you? It's an idea that's flourishing in some quarters, but you need to know where to look. My first book, *The Natural Advantage*, explores how organic farms are a model for work organisations. I compared some large businesses to battery chicken farms, and I stand by this; they're both exploiting living resources unsustainably. Big corporations and industrial farming are unlikely to disappear, but we can now see the organic alternatives thriving alongside them.

You're more likely to find community qualities in work organisations that are small or medium size: they could be charities, public sector bodies, social enterprises, or other kinds of value-based businesses. In the past 20 years, there's been rapid growth in social enterprise, which typically means using private capital and business disciplines to achieve social and environmental benefits, not profit. Terms like patient capital and impact investment describe funders who lend or invest money in social enterprises, and accept low financial returns because they believe in the mission.

All these kinds of organisation have qualities of community. Most of the people who work in them are there mainly because of the mission and values, not just to earn money. This means they're willing to challenge colleagues and "bosses" about such topics, and leading such a team is more like guiding a community than directing a for-profit company.

Community skills and values are urgently needed in mainstream society to help us all thrive in the pressures ahead, and work organisations are one way to help this. Few people will invest their own time to learn such skills, but I've seen them respond eagerly to workplace training on just these topics.

If you're involved with a work team that could develop as a community, learn all you can through this book and related resources, and then encourage colleagues to explore them too. You may want to avoid words like community, which could be alien to some people. Just seek support for goals like more effective meetings, and offer some practical steps towards them.

Profit and business are often seen as the villains of the climate crisis. This is part truth in a more complex situation; I prefer to support the views of American writer Paul Hawken. He sees the business sector as having the potential to reverse the climate crisis. As he says, business is not inherently destructive; it needs to operate by different rules (see more in Resources).

Resources

Community supported agriculture: for more info on how it works, plus case studies and project finder in the UK, see **http://www.communitysupportedagriculture.org.uk** For an international view, see **https://www.lowimpact.org**

The Hidden Life of Trees: by Peter Wohlleben. Written by a professional forester, this book combines a deep sense of trees as a living community with research evidence to support its views.

How everything can collapse: by Pablo Servigne and Raphael Stevens. A usefully sensible book on why and how our societies might collapse, and ways to reduce or respond to the risk, including the role of communities.

Seeding our Future: for more about the projects mentioned, and others, see **https://www.seedingourfuture.org.uk**

Future Conversations: for more about programme content, feedback and future events, see https://www.seedingourfuture.org.uk/future-conversations

Deep Adaptation: there is an extensive network of resources, discussion groups and more. Start with **https://www.deepadaptation.info**

Food security in Bridport: for progress reports, insights, newsletters and more, see **https://www.bridportfoodmatters.net**

Role models from Scotland: The New Road, by Alf and Ewan Young, is a delightful book — readable, informative, encouraging. It provides examples of community initiatives in a wide range of sectors, including housing, energy, food and more.

Woodland Immersions for Doctors: for more info, see https://www.seedingourfuture.org.uk and **https://hazelhill.org.uk**

Cohousing: for some introductory info, and a list of UK projects, see **https://cohousing.org.uk**, the website for the UK Cohousing Network. For more about sociocracy, see **https://www.sociocracyforall.org** or try a web search on this topic. There is a short case study on cohousing in Chapter 6.

Facing the 2020s: see more at **https://www.seedingourfuture.org.uk/adaptive-communities**

Community mapping: you'll find a detailed process and worksheets at **https://www.naturalhappiness.net/resources**

Communication skills: see Chapter 3 Resources for help with this.

Facilitation: for some basic guidelines, see *The Red Book of Groups,* by Gaie Huston. This is a short, simple book which covers a lot of essential points. *Facilitator's Pocketbook,* by John Townsend is a simple, practical primer on guiding groups, geared for work organisations, but relevant for other types of group too.

Group dynamics: try *Games People Play: the psychology of human relationships,* by Eric Berne. One of the classic books on this topic illuminating about group dynamics and one-to-one connections. *The Power of Us* by David Price is more geared to helping you improve dynamics within a group.

Conflict handling: See Chapter 3 for Resources.

Including fun and imagination: Rob Hopkins' book is *From What Is To What If: unleashing the power of imagination to create the future we want.*

Learning from intentional communities: Creating A Life Together, by Diana Leafe Christian. This book grows from decades of experience and dozens of communities. Whilst it's a how-to guide for starting an intentional community, the sections on community principles and dynamics are invaluable for all kinds of community, and the best book I know on the subject.

The Findhorn Book of Community Living, by Bill Metcalf. This shortish book gives you info on the history of intentional communities and specific projects.

The Ecology of Commerce, by Paul Hawken: this book shows how business is not inherently destructive of the planet or of people. As he points out, the business world has huge capabilities for positive change and regeneration if it is given the right ground rules, tax regime, etc.

Chapter 6

Growing through Climate Change

Gardeners can tell that climate change is a real problem: we see the droughts, gales and floods get worse each year. Tending the garden can be a haven of calm, a place to escape from the world's troubles. However, the climate crisis needs to be faced, and this chapter offers support.

I'm not going to spell out the alarming outlook: you probably know the gist, and if not, the Resources section can help you. My main aim is to offer ways to grow through difficult feelings like anxiety and bewilderment, to find your way to live with the ongoing crisis we're in, and see how you could make a positive contribution.

Human nature needs something to hope for, and that's hard to find when the outlook appears bleak. We need to redefine what kind of hope is possible, and to keep managing our perception of 'reality', because what we get through the media is a distorted picture, full of alarm, which we have to balance with other perspectives.

Probably many of us are living in overwhelm about climate change much of the time — or in denial, which is one way to cope with it. Stay aware of how much alarming information you can handle, and limit what you take in.

I hope this chapter enables you to prepare for the turbulent years ahead: to gather the skills of super-resilience, gain perspectives amid the confusion, and form a positive vision of how you'd like to grow, contribute, and be nourished. The first two sections are more about foundations, and the following two look at intention and direction. Imagine this is like preparing a garden for a tough spell (storms or drought). The foundations mean raising vitality and adaptability, clearing out problems. Then we'll explore intentions about how to meet challenges, and the outcomes you're aiming for. The four sections are:

Learning from Nature: insights and responses to the climate crisis, including the key concept of regeneration.

Frameworks and processes: approaches which can help you with difficult feelings, and with resilience.

Perspectives and big questions: ways to relate to climate change, and issues to consider.

Gathering your threads: suggestions to help you weave a way of being and acting through the years ahead.

Learning from Nature

The writer Thomas Berry says we need to feel for Nature the love a mother feels for a child. I reckon we need to feel the love a child has for its mother. When we speak of Mother Earth, it's not a figure of speech: Nature provides our food, water, and huge emotional nourishment.

Feeling this depth of love for our wounded planet may also connect us with pain and grief, and to some extent we need to. Usually love or pain motivate us to action, and it's clear that we need change on a massive scale. If we're strong enough to face the facts, Nature is showing us clearly the scale of the crisis we're all in. We know that humans are less motivated by preventing a negative outlook than by fulfilling a positive vision: face as much of the damage in Nature as you can cope with, but face it by picturing the damage reversed, and ecosystems thriving again.

Talkin' 'bout Regeneration

At present, both ecosystems and human systems (individuals and also support systems like healthcare) are depleted and overstressed. The essence of regeneration is to restore vitality and resilience, using natural processes where possible. One of the best examples of this approach is *regenerative agriculture* (RA): this means recovering the depth and fertility of topsoils, which in many places are depleted by soil runoff and use of chemicals. RA is well described in the website and books in Resources at the end of the chapter.

You could see regenerative agriculture as building on organic farming, but going further: one reason this is needed is that problems of soil erosion and fertility loss are so widespread and severe. Another reason is that it offers great potential for sequestering carbon from the atmosphere into the soil. Many plans for reducing the level of carbon in the atmosphere depend heavily on sequestering (i.e. removing) large volumes of CO_2 from the air. These plans usually assume this massive task will be achieved by technology, but *this technology is unproven as yet!* Hence RA could prove crucial.

Charles Eisenstein's book has a whole chapter on RA, explaining the principles, and with case examples. RA can involve closely controlled rotational grazing by livestock, and cover crops and perennial plants to avoid leaving soil exposed and at risk of erosion by rainwater runoff. Often multiple varieties of crops are grown together: the biodiversity helps control pests, and different root depths condition the soil.

Case Study: 2500 Acres of Regeneration in Buckinghamshire

Steve Lear farms 2500 acres on five sites in Buckinghamshire: in 2016 he realised that conventional farming methods were not working for him. The heavy clay was becoming very hard to work, yields were a problem, and advisers told him that his soil was dead. 'Of course, I then realised that I needed to change the whole system . . . so we ventured into cover crops, controlled traffic, muck management and including perennials in the rotation. We also started reducing inputs.' Changes include composting muck from his Limousin cows, mixing it with wood chip, and making it more biologically active. Including grass/clover in the rotation is another way of naturally improving fertility.

Steve has reduced or eliminated ploughing, and has not used insecticides for 3 years. 'Slugs are no worse than they were, and there's been no sign of the yield dip that some others have experienced.' He has also found that water runoff problems have reduced.

Adaptive Agriculture

This is another approach which gives grounds for hope. Many experts believe that disruption to food supplies will be the biggest climate impact for humans over the next decade and beyond. However, there's a lot of scope to adapt cultivation methods and crops to sustain output in new weather conditions.

As part of my food security project in Dorset, I commissioned a review of what adaptation will be needed in South West England. Here are some of the changes it highlights:

- A vital need is rainwater capture, to provide irrigation in droughts, and prevent soil runoff in heavy rains. This can be done through swales (drainage ditches) and ponds, ploughing along contour lines, etc.
- Mulching and intercropping (two or more crops grown together) can reduce both evaporation in hot periods and soil runoff in heavy rain.
- The crops grown will need to adapt to the warming climate: for example, apples, brassicas and swedes may struggle, but apricots, salads, maize will be more viable.

- Consumers can improve food security by diet changes, such as more beans and lentils, less meat. The UK produces plenty of wheat, but 40 per cent is used for animal feed.

Regenerative Agriculture to Regenerative Humanculture

How can we apply these parallels? It may help to consider that we humans are just as depleted as the earth by current habits. Soil is an organism with amazing powers of regeneration and resilience, providing we stop polluting it, and nourish it with natural energy sources. This is true for people too, and holding a vision of regeneration, of growing our vitality, can help motivate us to achieve it: the ways to do so are in this book.

However, we have to accept that the scale of the climate crisis is such that it won't be 'solved' in the next few decades. We are in an era where we have to adapt to disruptions and even collapse in both ecosystems and human systems. Related to the climate crisis is the accelerating loss of biodiversity: extinction and decline of many species of animals, birds, plants and more. The interactions between species are so complex and subtle that the impact of losses can't be forecast, including effects on human health, food supply and more.

This situation is sometimes compared to rivets on an aeroplane. The wings are held together by thousands of rivets. Clearly, you can lose a few without problems. At what point have so many rivets been lost that the plane crashes? When you face an uncertain threat, the best approach is the precautionary principle: this means, avoid taking any steps which could increase the risk. If you think about the systems of society generally, you can probably see many which are overstressed and suffering disruptions. What we can learn from the biodiversity crisis is that we can't forecast what degree of loss, what level of overload, will cause breakdowns, and that it can happen suddenly.

For many systemic problems, it's especially governments and businesses that need to apply the precautionary principle, but that doesn't look likely. However, local communities can start to create regenerative humancultures for themselves, and we can carry a vision of hope at this scale.

Frameworks and Processes

This section introduces you to approaches which have helped me relate to the climate crisis: they include ways to handle difficult feelings like fear and overwhelm, skills to raise your resilience, and methods to engage with the situation. There are books and websites about most of these approaches in Resources: this gives you a flavour, to decide if you want to explore further.

Active Hope

This is a book by Chris Johnstone and Joanna Macy. Here's the gist of what Active Hope means: this is the redefined kind of hope I mentioned at the start of the chapter.

Active Hope is a practice. Like tai chi or gardening, it is something we do rather than have. It is a process we can apply to any situation, and it involves three key steps. First, we take a clear view of reality; second, we identify what we hope for in terms of the direction we'd like things to move in or the values we'd like to see expressed; and third, we take steps to move ourselves or our situation in that direction.

Since Active Hope doesn't require our optimism, we can apply it even in areas where we feel hopeless. The guiding impetus is intention; we choose what we aim to bring about, act for, or express. Rather than weighing our chances and proceeding only when we feel hopeful, we focus on our intention and let it be our guide.

Chris Johnstone and Joanna Macy

Seeds of hope and the gardening metaphor can be useful here. When we plant actual seeds in the earth, we do so with love and care, we nourish them with water, and we accept that the outcome is uncertain: some of our planting will fail. This kind of faith is what Active Hope calls for. It also offers ways to understand our current situation, for example, the three 'stories of our time':

- *Business as Usual:* this is the story that governments and business would like us to believe. There's nothing basically wrong, and a bit more economic growth and technology will sort things out soon.
- *The Great Unravelling:* worsening climate change is only one of several huge problems which show that the world is falling apart and it's too late to save it.
- *The Great Turning:* whilst this story is less visible in the mass media it is already happening in many ways: tangible steps towards sustainability and regeneration.

To some extent, all three stories are happening, but only the third encourages us to act and believe we can make a difference. This book is also the most accessible way to explore Deep Ecology, covered below.

Deep Ecology: The Work That Reconnects

This is one of the best processes I've found to help face and move through the difficult feelings about the climate crisis which can easily push us into numbness or denial. It was created by Joanna Macy, one of the leading voices in the Deep Ecology field, which originates with Arne Naess. She comments:

> The cause of our apathy is not indifference. It stems from a fear of the despair that lurks beneath the tenor of life-as-usual . . .

Because of social taboos against despair and because of fear of pain, it is rarely acknowledged or expressed directly . . . The energy expended in pushing down despair is diverted from more creative uses, depleting the resilience and imagination needed for fresh visions and strategies. Fear of despair erects an invisible screen, filtering out anxiety-provoking data. In a world where organisms require feedback in order to adapt and survive, this is suicidal.

Joanna Macy

Her Work that Reconnects (WTR) approach combines ecology with Nature-based teachings from Buddhism and Native Americans. Joanna explains that this is a four-step cycle which we need to spiral round repeatedly, not as some one-off transformation. Let's explore each step briefly:

1. *Opening to gratitude.* Whatever your worries may be, shift your focus to thankfulness: for the gift of life, and all the resources that keep you alive. Include the many gifts of Nature, and the good things you receive from other people. Starting with gratitude helps us be present in the here and now, to relax and open up beyond our worries. As Joanna says: 'Thankfulness loosens the grip of the industrial growth society by contradicting its predominant message: that we are insufficient and inadequate. The forces of late capitalism continually tell us that we need more — more stuff, more money, more approval, more comfort, more entertainment.'

2. *Owning our pain for the world.* This stage can be tough: it helps to find a group or mentor to start it with. Most of us stuff down and deny the pain we feel about the Earth and its creatures being abused and destroyed. It takes courage to face your pain, and it can include a range of difficult feelings, such as anger, fear, guilt, despair, confusion. I've

led many groups through this process, and share Joanna's view that the key element is being able to voice your pain and have it witnessed by others. This breaks through the sense that these feelings are abnormal, and that you're alone with them.

3. *Seeing with new eyes.* By letting yourself feel your pain for the world, you open to a new sense of connection with it, and with other people who share our concerns. As individuals, we can feel powerless. When we feel ourselves part of the network of life, and part of a community, something different becomes possible.

4. *Going forth.* Macy describes this as 'the discovery of what can happen through us . . . one simply finds oneself empowered to act on behalf of other beings — or on behalf of the larger whole.' I'd add the idea of *being forth*, i.e. shifting our inner focus to a positive vision and qualities of trust and hope.

I highly recommend the WTR process, but advise you to use a trained, experienced facilitator who knows how to hold it.

Deep Adaptation

In Summer 2018, I was feeling that a quantum step-up in resilience was needed. Jem Bendell's Deep Adaptation approach offers this. Whilst Jem strongly supports all efforts to reduce climate change, he cites extensive evidence that it is too late to avoid serious worsening. He uses the term Deep Adaptation as a focus for facing and adapting to the adversities ahead, with four main aspects:

- **Resilience:** skills to handle deep emotions such as fear and grief. Facing the emotional impacts enables us to act more clearly and coherently. He endorses Deep Ecology as a good process for this.

- **Relinquishment:** letting go of behaviours and beliefs that prevent us adapting, for example around diet and travel, and what we feel entitled to.
- **Restoration:** recovering helpful approaches such as close-knit local communities.
- **Reconciliation:** this recognises that the pressures ahead may intensify polarities, extremism, scapegoating, and we need to get beyond them.

Jem believes that societal turmoil is likely in countries like the UK within the next 10 years. The most probable trigger is global food shortages. He shares the view of many experts that a Multi Bread Basket Failure is possible anytime from now: this means major crop failure in the same year for the few countries and staple foods that most of the world population depend on.

Jem also offers indicative ideas on how government and local communities can respond, including two ways we need to prepare for potential collapse, and find new skills and mindsets:

- *Collapse-readiness* includes the mental and material measures that will help reduce disruption to human life — enabling an equitable supply of the basics like food, water, energy, payment systems and health.
- *Collapse-transcendence* refers to the psychological, spiritual and cultural shifts that may enable more people to experience greater equanimity toward future disruptions and the likelihood that our situation is beyond our control.

I value how Jem acknowledges the emotional and spiritual impacts of facing a bleak outlook, and points to ways to process these, including faith, and 'a vision of people sharing compassion, love and play'. And he sees upsides and potential in what is likely to be a long period of major change.

Transformational Resilience

Transformational Resilience (TR) forms a valuable element in super-resilience, along with the other approaches in this section, and my Natural Happiness model. TR was created by an American, Bob Doppelt: his book is a good bridge between the global outlook and practical action, with an excellent array of self-help techniques.

I share Doppelt's view that we're now beyond the pattern of major crises followed by periods of normality. Continually rising disruption is more likely, and he argues that the mental wellbeing impacts will be extremely widespread, far beyond the capacity and methods of our mental health services. A key part of TR is his belief that trauma in response to the climate crisis is already widespread, and will grow further. What he offers in this book is a very well-researched approach, proven with many clients to cultivate transformational resilience: hopefully before our stress reaches trauma levels, but if necessary, after that.

Doppelt says, 'The psychological definition of trauma is that an experience seriously undermines or completely shatters at least some, if not all, of an individual's core assumptions and beliefs. . .climate disruption will produce this type of trauma for many.' He believes that many individuals, also organisations (such as health and other public services) and communities are already deeply affected by unresolved trauma. However, what he's advocating is not a massive process of therapy, but skills and processes to enable us to function better in a chaotic world.

His TR approach has two key aspects, and each has three core elements:

Presencing: 'the ability to deactivate and direct our psychological drives'
Ground: and centre yourself by stabilising your nervous system
Remember: your personal strengths, resources and social support network

Observe: your reactions to and thoughts about the situation non-judgementally with self-compassion

Purposing: 'the capacity to intensify the pull of meaning, direction, and hope in our lives'

Watch: for new insights and meaning in life and climate-enhanced hardships

Tap: into the values you want to live by in the midst of climate adversity

Harvest: hope for new possibilities by making choices that increase personal, social and environmental wellbeing

The book is designed for practical use: processes to enable these elements are described in detail, with self-help exercises, case studies and credentials of where they originated; for example, mindfulness. It offers a form of resilience which complements Jem Bendell's Deep Adaptation approach. Some adjustment from the USA context where Doppelt created this material will be needed for European readers; for example, because everyday levels of violence are much higher in the US.

Spiritual Ecology

The guiding thread in spiritual ecology is to regard the Earth as sacred and to see the environmental crisis as not just technical, but as reflecting humanity's loss of this sacred connection, and the feelings of love and responsibility that go with it. This viewpoint is being explored in political activism, in science, conservation, religion, and elsewhere.

This belief is held by many indigenous tribal cultures, and has been developed by various teachers over the past century. Thomas Berry is one of these, and we will explore his views in Chapter 7. The Buddhist monk Thich Nhat Hanh is another, who Jem Bendell recommends. A key aspect of spiritual ecology is the belief that all forms of life, including the Earth herself, are interconnected, in a web of interbeing.

So how can spiritual ecology help us as the climate crisis deepens? It can encourage us to lean away from a sense of isolation, and away from a hope (which government and business promote) that technology will save us. Instead, recognise that all life is in this crisis together, and we need the wisdom it offers: if humanity can truly listen to Nature and Gaia, and act upon what it hears, positive change can happen. In a recent blog, I wrote that for centuries, most human societies have put the needs and desires of the Masculine first, the Feminine second, and Nature third. If humanity is to survive, this has to be reversed; we have to give Nature the priority ahead of our own needs.

One of the articles I read while researching spiritual ecology quoted James Gustave Speth, a US Government adviser on climate change: 'I used to think that top environmental problems were biodiversity loss, ecosystem collapse and climate change. . .I was wrong. The top environmental problems are selfishness, greed and apathy, and to deal with these we need a cultural and spiritual transformation.'

Embodying the spiritual ecology approach takes more than a walk in the park. It needs immersion in Nature, and the will to challenge your assumptions. A deep link with a place where you can feel a sacred connection helps a lot, such as Hazel Hill Wood, and you can create this in your own garden.

Perspectives and Big Questions

In this section, we move from foundations to intentions. As you read on, see if you can shape your own view of the future outlook, and your priorities. What I'm sharing is not just my own reflections, but what I've gathered from a lot of contacts and research in recent years.

A Long View: Worse then Better

Sustainability issues have been on my radar for 40 years, and I've lived through a cycle where concern and hope reaches a peak, and ebbs away. This cycle has produced progress, but nowhere near enough. Where this leaves me is sadly doubtful that international bodies and national governments will enforce the drastic changes needed to keep global warming under 2 degrees. We can all see the short-term electoral pressures, vested interests, and other factors that have prevented rhetoric and reality on climate policies from converging for many years.

So what's ahead? My sense is that there will be continuing progress, but not enough, and that the climate crisis will get worse for many years, until around 2040. By this time, a tipping point could arise, leading to radical positive action by governments and societies across the world. This view is shared by Charles Eisenstein, one of the best-informed climate observers I know. Worse is likely to include more extreme weather events, food shortages, pandemics, refugee movements, and more.

The Precautionary Problem

This seems to be a fundamental issue in human psychology, which has been increasingly clear as I've tried to persuade my own local community to improve our food security. Many experts have observed that humans are designed to deal with tangible, immediate threats (like a woolly mammoth attacking), but struggle to respond to diffuse, complex, long-term issues.

Even if you feel there are future threats that need to be prepared for, you're likely to find that taking action is a problem. When no one else is acting, you may feel inhibited — do you want to go out on a limb? Many of the desirable preparations are at community level. How do you create collective momentum?

There are no easy answers to this, but there are clues and precedents. First, it's easier to gather people around a positive vision than a negative threat. Second, highlight issues that are more tangible, such as food or the local economy. Third, look for kindred spirits: this process is more sustainable with a few of you than alone.

Insights from Collapsology

A number of experts, including Jem Bendell, say that some form of societal collapse is likely within the next 10 years, so it's worth investigating this. What form of collapse, how temporary or long-term, and is it avoidable? The best resource I've found on these topics is a French book, by Servigne and Stevens, translated as *How Everything Can Collapse*. It's well-researched, and as constructive as one can be on a topic like this.

This book usefully explains different types or levels of collapse, and draws insights from ancient and modern collapses. They describe the model created by Dmitry Orlov with five progressively severe levels of collapse: financial, commercial, political, social, and then cultural: the latter meaning that 'faith in the goodness of humanity is lost'. There are now plenty of experts with gloomy views of the future, but it would help us all if they could clarify the degree of collapse they foresee, as that would guide us on ways to prepare for it.

Part II of the book is enticingly titled 'So, When's It Going to Happen?' This gathers a lot of useful data: both from quantitative models, and from analysts like Jared Diamond who have studied the causes of collapse in previous civilisations. Here are some of the insights:

- A collapse would arise from interaction of so many complex variables that its timing cannot be accurately predicted.
- Models of complex systems (natural and human) show that homogeneous and closely connected systems are more vulnerable, like the ones we have now.
- Several models of our current global system show that major income inequalities contribute substantially to the risk of collapse: the reasons why are well explained in the book, and are really worth understanding. They include the ways that wealthy elites are cushioned from crises

and slow to react, and how conspicuous consumption at the top orients most people towards emulating it.

- An updated version of the famous Club of Rome Limits to Growth model from the 1960s, done in 2004, predicts collapse from 2030 unless several drivers are all stopped: population growth, income inequality, and soil erosion/ agricultural crisis.

YOU HAVE NOW EARNED A SHORT INTERMISSION

This material is arduous, so award yourself a break. Go out in Nature, listen to soothing music, jump up and down and yell — whatever lets the tension out for you. Then have a small treat, and appreciate yourself. And relax and enjoy this cheerful picture.

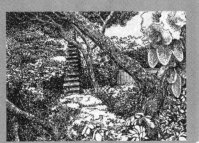

Crisis Events: Scenario Planning

Across the world, more and more people are being impacted by crisis events arising from climate change and other factors. The Precautionary Problem, described above, helps us to understand why public services, local communities and individuals are not as prepared as they could be. Consider exploring crisis events that could happen to you and your community, and ways you could prepare for them:

Scenario planning is a widely used method to do this. It involves envisaging a future event, picturing its consequences, and then considering what steps would reduce the impact if this event were to happen. Even if the event you imagine feels unlikely, this exercise can improve your skills in responding, and ability to act in an emergency. It's also a good community-building process.

One reason for doing this is to help you to think clearly and practically *about* an alarming situation, and hopefully *in* one if it happens. You'll need to draw on your resilience skills to carry this through. Probably your fears will come up: try to examine them to see which are valid, and which arise from old beliefs that you're projecting onto a future situation. To help you, here are some reassuring facts about typical crisis responses:

- The Servigne and Stevens book on collapse quotes a range of research about what actually happens, and concludes that: 'After a catastrophe. . .most human beings behave in extraordinarily altruistic, calm and composed ways.' Similar views on the caring and cooperative essence of human nature are well evidenced in the book by Rutger Bregman, *Humankind*. A lot of our fears arise from disaster movies and misleading media reports (for example, on Hurricane Katrina).
- In Britain, crisis events like floods have produced a positive response from communities, and so have terrorist bombing attacks.
- Even a breakdown of social order like the looting riots of 2011 in the UK did not lead to attacks on private individuals or people's homes.

The aim of a scenario review is to identify ways you can be more prepared for a crisis, and thus to raise your confidence and lower your anxiety. These ways include closer connection with neighbours and local community groups, prepping (discussed below), and your own resilience skills.

Prepping

This is a term for practical preparations for a crisis situation, such as emergency food supplies, and backup power and heating. It's a tricky topic, because some preppers take this to extremes. I don't see these as necessary, but there are simple steps anyone can take to provide some cover for the kind of crises described earlier. You can find more help with this in Resources.

Brain Mush and the Field of Fear

We know that for millennia, humans have reacted to crisis with fight, flight or freeze. A large, diffuse crisis such as climate change or a pandemic can't be fought with or fled from, so we can see a lot of apathy and confusion. On top of this comes what I call the field of fear: a collective feeling, which affects us all, but is hard to name and define. The crucial point here is to keep choosing your reality and your beliefs, and find some kindred spirits, otherwise you risk being sucked into this.

Technology vs. Nature, Big vs. Small

In our world, a lot of power rests with governments, large businesses, and institutions like the World Bank. Most of them feel some concern about climate change, but have other priorities which look bigger to them, and which limit the responses they can imagine. They want initiatives which are large-scale, controllable, and good for big business. This explains their focus on technology for vital issues like carbon sequestration, when soil cultivation has a better record so far.

As you weigh up how much hope to feel about the future, and what positive initiatives to support, both practically and in your prayers, widen your view beyond the rhetoric in the media. Look back at the description of Regenerative Agriculture, early in this chapter. E.F. Schumacher's famous book, *Small is Beautiful*, offers further encouragement. It could be that a myriad of labour-intensive organic farms will make the difference to carbon capture.

What About the Others?

In the troubles of recent years, it seems that most people's attention has focussed on their own situation, and their own country. There has been little reporting, even in the progressive media, of how badly this crisis is hitting economically poorer countries. Not only do many of these face a climate crisis of their own, they have also lost much of the human and financial aid that came in from Europe and America.

It's a tough truth to respond to, but we need to recognise that people in poorer countries are suffering bigger impacts from climate change, although they did less to cause it. This is yet another massive issue. I don't have any easy responses. At minimum, we can carry awareness of this issue in our hearts, we can share some of our resources, we can pray for the relief of suffering, picture a fairer sharing of resources globally, and support organisations in our own country which lobby for this.

A Soul Point of View

Have you ever tried imagining that all the rising turbulence of the climate crisis is a good thing, with positive outcomes? Here's another perspective to consider. In Chapter 7, I share my belief that we each have a soul, whose journey continues long before and after the human life we're in now. Imagine that your soul has chosen to be here on Earth during this crisis. Maybe there's something vital it can learn or contribute. Perhaps we're all here at this time to learn compassion and cooperation. This can be an empowering viewpoint to explore.

Sustainable, Sociable and Fun: A Cohousing Story

An ecological footprint is a measure of how much productive land area your lifestyle requires, and how far this is from sustainability. The UK average footprint is between 5 and

8 global hectares per person, based on different experts' views. This is a story of how simple measures at the cohousing project I co-founded achieved a carbon footprint of only 2.4 hectares per person.

In 2004, six of us bought an old farmhouse with outbuildings in North Dorset. We called our project the Threshold Centre: it was the first low-impact, affordable cohousing neighbourhood in the UK. Our sustainability plan addressed the three main sources of domestic carbon emissions:

- *Food:* we had a shared half-acre market garden, and group meals twice weekly reduced food waste.
- *Heating:* our planning permission to create a total of 14 dwellings (half affordable, funded by a housing association) included an efficient biomass boiler using wood pellets to heat the whole site.
- *Transport:* we minimised private car use, with social activities and play facilities on site, shared cars for outings and shopping. Households were limited to one private car each, and had to insure it as a pool car. This made it easy for a low-income household to avoid the cost of car ownership.

Try imagining the situation we may all face in a few years' time, when the cost of food and fuel could be much higher. You don't need a dedicated cohousing project to do this: you could set up simple sharing arrangements with others in your neighbourhood.

One of our guiding principles at the Threshold Centre came from Bill Dunster, the pioneering architect who set up the BedZED zero-emission housing scheme in London. He said, 'You have to make living sustainably more easy, and more fun, than a high emission lifestyle.' This community in Dorset continues to do just that.

Gathering the Threads

If you've read the chapter this far, well done! This stage is like the middle of the Diamond Process described in Chapter 4. Feeling a bit overloaded and confused is a good sign: give space for intuitions, imaginations and inspiration to come in. Going for a long walk, or relaxing with some music, can help this. This final section offers you pointers on how to find your focus, your intention, and start to fulfil it.

Find your passion, let it lead you: as you scan through ideas and possibilities, keep going until you find one or two where your spirits rise and your heart beats faster. Use the Diamond Process in Chapter 4 to help you explore an idea, see where it leads, and how to shape it into practical form.

Don't jump off the cliff — find the steps: sometimes when a big idea grips us, we think we have to throw our old life out the window. But there are exploratory steps you could start with, such as:

- Are there people or projects already doing something akin to your idea? Can you learn from them? (Chapter 5 has some good examples).
- Is there a way to test drive your fantasy? For example, work-shadow someone for a week, run a pop-up experiment or pilot project.
- Talk your idea over with a friend, create a 3-month groundwork plan to explore it.

Gather companions for the journey: for most initiatives, working with other people gives you more wisdom, skills and support.

*Value being **and** doing:* in mainstream society, it looks like only action counts. The climate crisis demands action, but that's not all. Realise how your presence, your beliefs, your prayers can be a gift.

See where you can support others: sometimes our best role is not to lead the charge, but to help existing projects. Be discerning about what's needed. It might be practical tasks, but also appreciation, encouragement, and witnessing other people's commitment.

The Love in Deep Adaptation: these parting words bring us back to the theme of Active Hope, near the start of this chapter. The reality of the years ahead is likely to be growing turmoil, with a risk of rising distress. So what can we realistically hope for? The passage below is from a blog by Jem Bendell, called The Love in Deep Adaptation.

One thing that rapid climate change can help us to learn is the destructiveness of our delusions about reality and what is important in life. Key to this delusion is the emphasis many of us place on our separate identities. Since birth, this othering of other people and nature means we dampen any feelings of connection or empathy. Seeking physical and psychological security and pleasure through control of our surroundings and how people interact with us is both a personal malaise and at the root of our collective malaise.

It is easier to consider other people's pain as less valid as one's own pain or that of the people and pets we know. But there is another way. The suffering of others presents us with an opportunity to feel and express love and compassion. Not to save or to fix, but to be open to sensing the pain of all others and letting that transform how we live in the world. It does not need to lead to paralysis or depression, but to being fully present to life in every moment, however it manifests. This approach is the opposite of othering and arises from a loving mindset, where we experience universal compassion to all beings. It is the love that our climate predicament invites us to connect with. *It is the love in deep adaptation.*

Jem Bendell

Resources

Regenerative agriculture: The website **https://regenerationinternational. org** gives a useful overview.

Climate: A New Story by Charles Eisenstein. Provides perceptive insights on the issues, and encouraging, well-researched antidotes, including regenerative agriculture.

Farming on the Wild Side by Nancy and John Hayden. This is an inspiring, detailed account of a regenerative farm in the US, which will give you a vivid picture of practical methods you can adapt to human regeneration.

Adaptive agriculture: The report by Elise Wach, *Growing through Climate Change*, is available in the food and farming section of my website, **https://www.seedingourfuture.org.uk**

Active Hope: this book is co-authored by Joanna Macy and Chris Johnstone. You can see more about Chris's books, events, etc. at **https://chrisjohnstone.info**. His book *Find Your Power* is also very helpful.

Deep Ecology: A good overview is the book *Deep Ecology: living as if Nature mattered*, by George Sessions and Bill Duval.

The Work that Reconnects: The book *Active Hope* is a good introduction. For fuller briefing on the process, see *Coming back to life: the updated guide to the Work that Reconnects*, by Joanna Macy and Molly Young Brown. See also **https://www. joannamacy.net** and **https://workthatreconnects.org**

Deep Adaptation: if you do a web search on these words, you'll find a range of websites, forums and other online resources, including **https://www.deepadaptation.info** and **http:// deepadaptation.ning.com**

Post Doom, No Gloom: Michael Dowd offers a lot of useful resources on how to adapt to the alarming outlook we face. Those include video conversations with many wise experts, and teaching videos with topics like Essential Wisdom for Hard Times and Reality 101. See **http://www.postdoom.com**

Transformational Resilience: the book is by Bob Doppelt. The related website is **http://www.theresourceinnovationgroup.org**

Spiritual Ecology: for books, try *Spiritual Ecology: 10 Practices to Reawaken the Sacred in Everyday Life,* by Llewellyn Vaughan-Lee, or *Spiritual Ecology: The Cry of the Earth,* a collection from writers including Joanna Macy, Thich Nhat Hanh and others. St Ethelburga's in London offers trainings and workshops, see **http://www.stethelburgas.org**

A Long View: if you want an informed view of the future outlook, try these books: *The Precipice,* by Toby Ord, or *The Uninhabitable Earth,* by David Wallace-Wells. Be warned, these books are alarming. The book *How Everything can Collapse* is more digestible, by Servigne and Stevens. You can see an excerpt at **https://www.resilience.org**

Prepping: Most books on this topic are American, and may strike British readers as overly paranoid. Best to read them selectively and with a large pinch of salt. For a very basic UK guide, see *Prepping in the UK* by S. Miller. Or try *Prepper Supplies and Survival Guide,* from Novato Press, or *The Prepper's Pocket Guide,* by Bernie Carr. There's also plenty of information on websites.

Technology vs. Nature, Big vs. Small: You may find E.F. Schumacher's celebrated book relevant: *Small is Beautiful.*

Ecological footprint: a web search will provide a range of briefing and estimates of global and national footprints, and ways to estimate your own footprint. There are differing calculation methods, which is one reason why figures for the UK range between 5 and 8 hectares per person. You can see more about the Threshold Centre at **http://www.thresholdcentre.org.uk**

The Love in Deep Adaptation: if you web search this blog title you should find it at **https://jembendell.com**

Chapter 7

Natural Inspiration

This chapter explores how you can access insights and resources by connecting with qualities like vision, higher consciousness, and soul. I'll share ways of doing this that work for me, many of them linked to Nature and the garden.

The future outlook for all of us is turbulent. We're going to need a quantum step up in our resilience, and that's what this chapter aims to offer you. I believe the fastest way to do this is by a deeper connection with inspiration, and what we might call higher dimensions. These need to be woven into your engagement with everyday physical and emotional realities, and gardening can show us how to do this.

Some of the approaches in this chapter may seem strange or esoteric. It's up to you to decide what may be useful for you. All the methods described are ones I've used for several years or more, but some of them took a good deal of practice or training. If you want to use them, it may need time and patience. The Resources section has pointers on this.

The first main section of the chapter, Inspiration with the garden, introduces some of the topics we'll explore in later sections. The next describes specific methods I use for natural inspiration, such as attunement. The third main section reviews ways to access and sustain inspiration, such as soul connection, self-care practices, and a faith path. The fourth section explores ways to apply inspiration, in shaping a vision and recovering from setbacks.

Inspiration with the Garden

As far as possible, I'm writing this book in our garden, and with the garden. My hope is that some of Nature's wisdom flows through me. Research confirms that our awareness expands in Nature, we relax out of screen world and open to new possibilities. So if you can, read this section in a garden, or at least imagine you're in one, and that we're exploring together.

As I look around the garden, I feel uplifted by its abundance, beauty and generosity. So many different plants, each with its own leaf, flower, fruit and so on. Look closely at some flowers or fruits, smell a rose. Is all this just physical, merely the result of evolution? Gardens lead me to believe that there is a bigger creative power at work, which I would call divine: a higher, non-physical dimension. When I need to give this power a name, I call it divine unity, because I believe it exists in every form of life — plants, animals, humans, and in the earth itself.

The poet Dylan Thomas wrote these lines:

The force that through the green fuse drives the flower
Drives my green age; that blasts the roots of trees
Is my destroyer

This is the presence I feel in the garden, which I call divine unity. Often the first line of this poem is quoted without the next two, but we have to accept that if there is some greater power in our world, it includes both creation and destruction, growth and decay. The garden reminds us that all this is part of Nature, and we need to include both in our human lives too.

Being in the garden helps me to expand awareness beyond my individual focus, and feel part of divine unity. It also keeps me humble: indoors with my smartphone or laptop, I can be suckered into thinking that humans control their world. Out here, I believe in something bigger, and it's easier to move into dialogue with that greater power.

The literal meaning of inspiration is to take in spirit or breath: in many languages there's only one word to mean both. When I breathe in the garden, I feel a strong connection to a bigger source, which could be called spirit. This is how I often receive new ideas, solutions to challenges, and a sense of nourishment.

Another idea I connect with in the garden is soul. Like many words in this chapter, it can be used in various ways: for me, soul is the piece of divine essence within each life, not just in people. As the Sufi teacher Inayat Khan puts it, 'Not only the living creatures but also trees and plants, and planets and stars, everything that exists has a spirit at the back of it, and that spirit is its soul.' In the garden, I relate more easily with my own soul, and with the divine essence in all life. It's like a spirit-level version of the worldwide web.

Going Deeper with Nature

This section invites you to explore some of the processes I use to engage more closely with the wisdom and power of the natural world.

Attuning with the Garden *Devas*

Much of my learning about inspiration and Nature comes from the Findhorn Foundation, an ecovillage and spiritual community in Scotland. Attunement is their word for a form of meditation where you tune in and align yourself with a source of guidance, including Nature, and with a project or work team. Attuning with devas has been a core part of Findhorn Foundation's philosophy for over 50 years, and I've been using it since I first went there in 1990. Its benefit is deeper dialogue with the intelligence of Nature, and scope to align your needs with those of a garden, or any other project. Machaelle Small Wright is an American who trained at Findhorn and took this further in creating her Perelandra garden in Virginia.

You begin an attunement with commitment to listening and serving the highest good of the garden, project or situation. With this intent, you then call in other presences or guides, such as the *devas*. A range of people, not just Findhorn, use *deva* to mean the living consciousness within a species of plants, in a whole garden, or in other forms of life. This is a very simple version of complex ideas: see Resources for ways to understand it in more depth.

A *deva* (pronounced *day-va*) could be described as the guiding consciousness of a place, project, or plant family, such as tomatoes or jasmine. The idea of a dialogue with an intangible presence like this may sound bizarre to you. The experience at Findhorn, and in our garden and many others, suggests that it has tangible benefits.

Here's an example. Linda and I see ourselves as co-creating our garden with the living presences of the plants and the land. When we wanted to erect a polytunnel, we went out and opened an attunement with the *deva* of the garden. We explained our intention and why we needed to do this, and listened for the voice of the garden, to understand its needs. As a result, we chose a different location from our first idea, one which has worked very well.

We also use attunement for everyday gardening decisions. For example, how to germinate parsnips, which is notoriously tricky. Asking for help from the Parsnip *Deva*, we were advised to sow seeds in the greenhouse in biodegradable pots which could be planted out straight into an outside bed. The result was a magnificent crop, compared to repeated failures the year before.

Over the years in our garden, we've had several situations with what you might call pests: such as slugs, wasps and moles. We start by attuning with the *deva* of the species, and aiming to negotiate. We do as Findhorn advise: explain our needs, ask for the response we'd like, and *offer an alternative option*. You need to accept that these creatures are part of your garden, and offer them another location, or something else to feed on. This approach usually works, but occasionally we've had to intervene, after warning them of our intention.

The attunement process can be used to work co-creatively with the guiding spirit of a project, a relationship, or a team. At Findhorn, I love volunteering for a shift in the kitchen: to start, the cooking crew join hands in a circle, and set their intention to create a wonderful meal. If I'm working with more mainstream groups, I adapt the process, having a minute of silence to 'tune in' to the highest good of the situation, and the best possible outcome.

Machaelle has also evolved a method called the coning meditation, to balance guidance from Nature with human wishes in all kinds of situations, from personal health to major projects. I have used it for 30 years, including writing this book. See more in Resources.

Case Study: Attunement in Action — the Forest Ark

The project where I've used attunement most consistently for many years is Hazel Hill Wood. Experience here confirms that it takes a while to establish connections between humans and *devas*, and this improves the longer you continue.

Hazel Hill is a conservation woodland and retreat centre, so any new building implies considerable disruption, especially as we fell our own timber to use in construction. The idea of a new structure never arises from an audit of needs, it slowly grows like a seed, from listening to the wood and to the people most involved with it.

In 2007, the concept of a new building was like a bud, or small seedling. We had a core group meeting at the wood, and attuned to this possibility. We called in the *deva* of the wood, along with the Angel of the human project at Hazel Hill, and the Angel of stewardship, as the quality which could help us balance human needs with the many other forms of life we share this space with.

We began our process at one of the trees we have sat with and talked with many times. Our experience is that certain trees are more open to dialogue with people and will relay such conversations to the community of trees in the wood. We left pauses in the conversation so that the gatekeeper tree could take in and share our suggestions and questions.

The response we felt from the wood was positive about a new building, but with several conditions. It should be an off-grid, low-impact building, both for the sake of the wood, and as a teaching aid with visitors. It should look as if it had grown from the wood organically. And it should use a lot of our own timber, lovingly shaped by craftspeople.

This became the brief for the Forest Ark building, which is amazing — check out pictures on the Hazel Hill website. One vital part of our attunement was to choose the location for the building, and to prepare the land, plants and wildlife for the forthcoming disruption, explaining our reasons for the new structure, asking for tolerance.

Another major attunement task was preparing the wood for a significant felling programme. The frame of the Ark needed us to fell 20 mature oak trees. Our forester identified and numbered 28 candidates: we sat and attuned with each one to see which were willing to be transformed and which wanted to stay.

Something we've learned from this and other felling work is that you need to prepare the remaining, standing trees as much as those to be cut. There is major shock for all of them, and we've used attunements after the felling to help clear it.

The Dream of the Earth

Although I've been raising my resilience to respond to climate change for several years, I still hit a sense of gloom most weeks. There are two teachers I turn to in my low points. One is Joanna Macy, whose Deep Ecology process was presented in Chapter 6. But if I hit rock bottom I turn to Thomas Berry, who wrote *The Dream of the Earth* and other books. Berry described himself as a cosmologist and Earth Scholar — he comments that not only does materialist society regard the planet as something to be used, but also our culture sees humans as separate from the Earth and other life on it. He was one of the early advocates of spiritual ecology, described in Chapter 6.

Berry writes passionately of the Earth and the universe as living, intelligent entities with their own evolutionary path. He co-wrote *The Universe Story* with physicist Brian Swimme: there were many points in its history where survival and progress were so improbable that it's more likely a guiding wisdom was involved.

He believes that *myth* is at the root of both the problem and the solution: 'The main difficulty in replacing the industrial order is not the physical nature of the situation, but its mythic entrancement. . .the myth is primary. . .so far the energy evoked by the ecological vision has not been sufficient to offset the energies evoked by the industrial vision — even when its desolation becomes so obvious. . .

Berry coined the term The New Story, to describe the vision, dream, myth we need to animate us. It's crucial to the new story that we humans see ourselves as part of the continuing Story of creation. Deeper contact with Nature can give us the insights to move forward, and the passion to act on them. As Berry says, 'Tough though it may be, we need to intensify our love for the Earth, and our sense of its pain, to motivate the radical changes humans need to make. This reenchantment with the Earth as a living reality is the condition for our rescue of the Earth from the impending destruction we are imposing on it.'

Berry has a feeling of optimism about the future, which continues to surprise and encourage me. It arises from his sense of the intelligence of Gaia, and a belief that if Gaia allowed humans to create this mess, it must be a huge growth opportunity for both humans and the planet:

The basic mood of the future might well be one of confidence in the continuing revelation that takes place in and through the earth. If the dynamics of the universe. . .guided us safely through the turbulent centuries, there is reason to believe that this same guiding process is precisely what has awakened in us our present understanding of ourselves and our relation to this stupendous process.

Thomas Berry

Going Higher with Inspiration

This section shares some of the ways I connect with inspiration which are not directly Nature-related. They are part of my approach to sustaining resilience and seeking insights amid the growing confusion of our times.

Soul Connection

The term soul clearly has resonance for many people: we talk about heart and soul, soul mates, and more. If you find the word difficult to engage with, imagine instead that I'm talking about essence. My belief about soul is that it's a piece of divine consciousness, present in all forms of life, but with different levels of awareness. I reckon that plants, trees and animals have a soul, but don't expect to have the same depth of dialogue with them as with a human soul.

I believe that human souls exist long before and after a human lifetime, and that they choose beforehand each incarnation they come into. This outlook helps me hugely when I hit a challenge: instead of feeling like the victim of random fate, I start from the view that my soul has *chosen* this situation for its own development. All I have to do is figure out what it wants to learn, and how!

The nearest thing I've found to objective evidence for this belief is the book *Journey of Souls* by Michael Newton (see more in Resources). He was an American hypnotherapist, who discovered that he could enable clients to connect with their soul at the time before it incarnated. His book shows how hundreds of clients independently reported the same features of the soul's journey. For example, that souls have learning clusters with a shared focus: these are the soul's home community, and several souls from a cluster may choose connected human lives as friends or family, so they can support each other.

I seek a dialogue with my soul most weeks. Sometimes I also try to set up a soul-level conversation with the soul of a work team, a project, a garden or a relationship. This can help to give a higher perspective on a situation, which gets above the personality or ego level (in you *or* other people!)

If you want to seek a soul connection yourself, start by choosing a congenial space: somewhere peaceful and supportive, out in Nature, or an indoor meditation space. And be patient: ask for a connection with your soul, but realise that it may take time for your soul to respond, and communication might be very brief and simple at first. Calling in a guide can help this connection: see more on this below.

Invisible Guides and Helpers

One of my beliefs is that there are many more levels of existence than we humans are usually aware of. These higher or subtler levels are hard for us to understand fully, but there are ways to access them and get support and guidance from them. The earlier section on working with *devas* is an example. If the idea of getting help from higher, intangible levels sounds possible to you, try exploring it in any way that comes to you intuitively.

If you have friends who do this, ask what works for them. Here are a few of the approaches which have helped me:

- Calling for guidance from a teacher in one of the spiritual traditions, such as Buddha, Jesus, Green Tara, Moses, Kwan Yin.
- Asking for help from a teacher you have met and worked with, or one where you feel a connection through books or videos.
- Connecting with an Angel who embodies a particular quality you need. This might be an Archangel, such as Raphael for healing. Or use the Angel cards created at Findhorn, and draw one at random to see what quality can help you best.
- Praying for help. You might pray to divine unity with whatever name you prefer, or to a saint, *bodhisattva*, or other presence who embodies a particular form of support you need. It's important to pray for outcomes that serve the greater good, not just your own needs, and to let go of any attachment to results (see Resources for more on this).
- Drawing on Nature connection. I often ask for support and guidance from the big ash tree in my garden, or from the *deva* of Hazel Hill Wood. Or you could call on Pan, who Machaelle and others see as the divine presence who oversees the natural world.

Inspirational Self-Care

There are so many pressures which can pull us into a state of brain mush, a feeling of isolation and helplessness. This is the 'normal' atmosphere we live in, reinforced by social media, news, fake news, domineering governments and more. We have to make repeated choices to maintain our power to discern and act for ourselves, and to sustain our positive connection with other people.

At the start of this chapter, I wrote of the need for a quantum step-up in our resilience. To achieve this, and maintain it, we need to make time frequently for self-care on the inspirational level. Here are some of the main methods I use:

- *Daily meditation and prayer:* I start every day with half an hour of meditating, and 5 minutes of prayers. This means that I start most days feeling calm, well grounded and resilient. It's also a time to set my intentions for the day, and to pray for help with issues at all levels, from personal to global.
- *Gratitude:* frequently giving thanks for whatever is positive, in our own lives and more widely, is a good way to raise your energy and antidote the pervading, disempowering bad news around us.
- *Visualising positive outcomes:* energising a vision of a positive outcome is more motivating and animating than trying to react to a negative outlook, and I believe it helps to bring a hope to actuality.
- *Embodiment, sound and movement:* I've found that these are powerful ways to deepen my connection with divine spirit, and to respond with resilience to setbacks. What I mean by embodiment is various ways to infuse my physical body with inspiration and positive emotions like gratitude. Sound mantras, chanting, devotional dance and walking meditation are some of the methods I use: see Resources for more information.
- *Ration your attention:* long periods online and on social media keep us anxious, disempowered, unable to concentrate. Many experts advocate limiting your exposure to the news and social media, and I've found this makes a big difference.

Faith, Hope and a Spiritual Path

The medieval Sufi teacher Ibn Arabi said, 'For hope you need faith,' and it's just as true today. In recent years, there have been many research studies on the factors which help people to be more resilient and adaptable. These show that people with a faith framework or spiritual practice are on average more cheerful, and recover better from setbacks of all kinds. I'm aware that this can be a delicate and personal topic for many people, but I'd like to offer some suggestions on how faith can help us, and how to explore this.

For me, the essence of faith is trusting in a power which can't be measured or understood logically. And to be honest, if I didn't have faith that there is some power greater than human greed, I'd despair. In fact, I believe that human love is more powerful than greed, and divine love and wisdom is more powerful still. Although it's often hard, I keep faith that there is some higher purpose even in suffering, and that we can reach out in prayer and ask for help for ourselves and others.

What I mean by a spiritual path is ongoing beliefs and practices which help to give you some hope and steadiness amid the alarms and uncertainties of life. Such a path could be a recognised framework like Buddhism or Christianity, but it doesn't need to be. I have gardener friends whose path is simply wordless communion with their garden, whose faith is rooted in the way that the Earth keeps giving and forgiving.

My spiritual path draws on Nature, and on some of the faith traditions, and I want to describe it here, in case it is of help to you. The unifying strand is a Sufi one. There are many flavours of Sufism, but it's not a religion: there's no one teacher, no creed, no temples. I view the essence of the Sufi approach as seeing divine essence in all forms of life, and accepting that divine unity is beyond human comprehension, it truly is a matter of faith from the heart.

Another strand is Aramaic Christianity, which is pretty different from church religion. For many years I've followed the teachings of Neil Douglas-Klotz, who has re-translated Jesus' teachings from Aramaic, the language Jesus spoke. This gives a much more deep, compassionate, empowering quality to them. And a further strand is Buddhism, which Jem Bendell also finds helpful in adapting to the climate crisis.

If the idea of a spiritual path calls to you, I suggest you start a process of exploration, preferably with some in-person groups and teachers, as well as books and online. And remember that Nature is one of our best spiritual guides!

Applied Inspiration: Visions and Recovery

This section considers how to apply inspiration to big issues in your life: in particular by forming a vision of what you're seeking, and in recovering from a major setback. Many studies show that people who have a sense of direction and inspiration about their life are more resilient generally. The guidelines below can help you create a vision for your life as a whole or any aspect of it, including your garden!

- **Explore different needs.** Firstly, understand your personal needs, including emotional (support, belonging etc.), practical (agreeable home, enough money and so on) and work-related, such as doing something worthwhile and being recognised. Then consider the needs of people close to you, and wider issues that you care about.
- **Listen to the land.** Many people find that this is just as helpful in planning their own lives as in planning a garden.
- **Set a time horizon.** This can help you to consider major trends which could affect you in future, also the longer-term effects of changes you make now.
- **Understand your basic constraints.** This means being realistic about your temperament — what aspects

of life and work nourish you or get you down? And being realistic about constraints such as your health, commitments, money needs, so that you shape a vision which is attainable.

- **Take time, use different approaches.** These might include some structured time in Nature, reading a self-help book, doing a few things which really inspire you, and talking things through with a friend.
- **Keep it flexible.** As with your garden, be pragmatic about how you apply your overall aims and principles, and review your progress regularly.
- **Aim for the highest good.** You may find a number of tensions between different needs as you try to create a vision for yourself, so use this principle to find the best overall outcome.
- **Walk for meaning.** This is a walk where you set an intention at the outset, and then spend one to six hours walking in Nature, open to whatever insights arise.

Recovery from a Major Setback

In these stormy times, we have to be resilient to big upsets as well as everyday ones, in our lives and in our gardens, and natural inspiration can help with this. Here are some pointers which can help in both of these:

- *Look after yourself:* there's probably some shock and grief about a big loss. Give yourself time to rest, to compost the feelings, and get some support.
- *Reconnect with your vision:* this is a way of getting some perspective on the setback. Feel what inspires you about your overall hopes, and your longer timeframe, to offset the loss. Accept that you may need to review and revise your vision to learn from this situation.

- *Be co-creative, seek the upside:* setbacks in the natural world generally have a positive aspect too. For example, if a gale flattens a beautiful mature tree, it creates an opening for new growth. With other problems, the benefits may be harder to find, but use your co-creative skills to seek them.
- *Listen to the garden:* with a sudden large problem, you probably need some new, different insights. Try sitting in the garden and asking for them, perhaps in the wild margins.
- *Take action:* don't get stuck in negative feelings or fretful thoughts. Keep yourself well rooted by doing something practical, even on a small scale: your best ideas may happen this way.

We're now at the end of our journey together: I wish you well with your future, and I hope this book provides ongoing help. If you'd like to keep in touch, you can easily do so via my website, newsletter and events. Let's remember how Nature will keep nourishing and guiding us if we keep choosing to reconnect.

Resources

Attuning with devas: The fullest account of this approach at Findhorn is the book *The Findhorn Garden*, which has chapters by the key figures from the founding of the project. For a detailed, practical guide to working with *devas* and other subtle energies in your garden, see the *Perelandra Garden Workbook,* by Machaelle Small Wright, aptly subtitled A Complete Guide to Gardening with Nature Intelligences. Her website is **https://www.perelandra-ltd.com**

Coning Meditations: There is a concise guide to the process and how to use it with your garden in Chapter 18 of the *Perelandra Garden Workbook.*

The Dream of the Earth: by Thomas Berry. This offers you perspectives on humanity's relationship with Nature, and the role of vision, dream and myth in engaging with the climate crisis. He also co-wrote *The Universe Story* with the physicist Brian Swimme.

Soul Connection: The book I recommend is *Journey of Souls* by Michael Newton, **https://www.newtoninstitute.org** See also *Testimony of Light* by Helen Greave, which is a detailed account of the afterlife, transmitted from a dead nun to a living one. . .

Praying for help: a good format for releasing attachments to outcomes is the Pink Bubble Technique in the book *Creative Visualisation* by Shakti Gawain.

Embodiment, Sound and Movement: this is a big topic, and it is ideal to explore this experientially through workshops and live groups. My main teacher in this area has been Neil Douglas-Klotz; find out more at **https://abwoon.org**. The form of devotional dance I have found most powerful is Dances of Universal Peace: see more at **http://www. dancesofuniversalpeace.org.uk**

Spiritual paths: a good starting guide is William Bloom's book, *The Power of Modern Spirituality*, not linked to any one path. His website is also useful: **http://www.williambloom.com**

Exploring Sufism: Idries Shah's books are one way in, e.g. *The Sufis or The Way of the Sufi*, or the wonderful novel by Reshad Feild, *The Last Barrier*. Or see *The Sufi Book of Life* by Neil Douglas-Klotz. For online and in-person groups, see **https:// inayatiyya.org**

Aramaic Christianity: see Neil Douglas-Klotz's books, especially *Prayers of the Cosmos*.

Appendix:
Resource Toolkit

This Appendix provides some longer processes and briefings to help you put Natural Happiness into practice. Some are in this Appendix, some are on the related website: **https://www. naturalhappiness.net/resources.** They are listed below by the chapter they relate to:

Chapter 2: Personal Energy Audit, Appendix
Chapter 3: Conflict Resolution Process, website
Chapter 4: Circle of Voices, Appendix
Chapter 5: Facing the 2020s: community insights, Appendix
Chapter 5: Community mapping process, website
Chapter 7: Embodiment, sound and movement, website

Personal Energy Audit
Assess your energy inflows and outflows — physical, emotional, mental inspirational — and see how to balance them.

When professionals assess the sustainability and resilience of many systems, they use an energy audit. This lays out the sources of energy, the processes which use it, and the outputs of the system. These audits are used for ecosystems, and also in designing buildings. I've adapted this idea to create a Personal Energy Audit, to help you see where your energy comes from, and how it's used. Most energy audits are calculated with measurable units like kilowatts: this one relies on your estimates.

Use the checklist below to assess the main energy inflows and outflows in your life and work. The processes in which you *use* energy should be considered as outflows. The items listed are not meant to be comprehensive: add others that are significant to you. For each one, rate its importance on a scale of 0 (low energy flow) to 10 (highly important, major energy flow). As you go through, put an asterisk in the Review Priority column for items you feel need most consideration. Remember that some items may be both a source and use of energy.

Initially, do these ratings for your current lifestyle and way of working: then you may wish to do the exercise again, to see how much impact a different approach or a new job would have. Also, remember that outflows include both useful ones, and those that 'waste' your energy.

When you have finished the audit, add your inflow and outflow scores for each of the four energy types, then total them. If you are running an energy surplus, congratulations! If you are running an energy deficit, ask yourself what's causing this. Look at items you asterisked for attention. Choose up to five of these as current priorities. How would you like your energy habits to change in these areas, and how might you set about making a change?

When you start to draw on natural energy sources and manage your ecosystem consciously, use the Personal Energy Audit as a way of measuring your progress and steering your priorities. It can also help you evaluate major decisions about your job or lifestyle in advance.

Circle of Voices

This is a method I've evolved for integrating multiple viewpoints: see Chapter 4 for a fuller introduction. Before you do this process, read this briefing thoroughly, and get clear on basic decisions such as aim, location, and who's involved. Set aside more time than you estimate — this doesn't work if you're in a hurry!

Aim: it's best to set this a couple of days beforehand, so your subconscious and intuition can prepare. Listen receptively for the outcome you'd like: don't push it or apply willpower. Your aim could be a broad, open question, such as 'to understand my best response to situation X', or it could be very specific.

Use this checklist to assess the main energy inflows and outflows in your work and life generally: rate each item from 0 (unimportant) to 10 (very important). Use the third column to highlight priorities for further review.

PHYSICAL	Energy Inflow	Energy Outflow	Review Priority
Everyday activities (e.g. work, commuting, housework)			
Diet: 'healthy' sustaining food/drink 'unhealthy' food/drink			
Breathing (deeper, relaxed is energizing)			
Exercise			
Relaxation			
Time in nature			
Indulgences (alcohol, smoking etc.)			
Other:			
SUBTOTAL			

	Energy Inflow	Energy Outflow	Review Priority
EMOTIONAL			
Self-appreciation or put-down: supporting or blaming yourself			
Appreciation or negativity from family and friends			
The emotional rewards or pressures of your job content and work organisation			
Support, challenges from your local community, neighbours etc.			
How do you respond to unexpected changes? Are they typically a stimulus or a stress for you?			
Emotional support/demands from any groups you are part of			
The emotional rewards or demands of your leisure time/hobbies			
Other:			
SUBTOTAL			
MENTAL			
Does your work and lifestyle give you mental stimulus or exhaustion?			
Do your family, friends, time with groups give you mental stimulus or exhaustion?			
Does the team/organisation you work in give you mental stimulus or depletion?			
Is your habitual way of thinking positive and creative, or do you tend to worry and fret and focus on the negatives?			

144

	Energy Inflow	Energy Outflow	Review Priority
Do you use both logical and intuitive skills and integrate them?			
Do uncertainty and conflicting data stimulate or dissipate your mental energy?			
Do you have leisure activities that give you mental energy or depletion?			
Other:			
SUBTOTAL			

INSPIRATIONAL

	Energy Inflow	Energy Outflow	Review Priority
Do you have a sense of purpose and inspiration in your life generally?			
Do you have a mentor, friend or teacher, or colleague who is a role model for you in connecting with inspirational energy?			
When life or work gets exhausting, can you re-energize yourself by remembering the point of it all?			
Does your view of the world and future outlook depress or uplift you?			
In your free time, do you choose any activities that inspire you (e.g. through nature, music, meditation), or do you choose distractions or compensations for stress and fatigue?			
Do you get inspiration from contact with Nature?			
Other:			
SUBTOTAL			
GRAND TOTAL			

Location: you need to do this process in a congenial setting where you won't be disturbed. Outside in Nature works best for me: an evening with a campfire is a good option if possible.

Who's involved: I've written the process assuming you're doing it alone. If you have one or more people to do it with, this can deepen the process. Here are some ways you could adapt it to include others:

- With one other person, ask them to give you general support, to offer any intuitions, name other voices that need hearing, and to speak for some of those voices if they feel a calling to do so.
- With two or more people, pause occasionally during the process to get their insights and suggestions; you might ask them to represent some of the voices, or invite them to propose voices who need including.

If you're working with others, tell them your aim for the session, give them a short briefing on the situation you're exploring, but don't make this too detailed. When someone steps into a role or a voice, some kind of intuition often guides them, and you may get insights you could never have expected. If you're guiding the process yourself, I'd only work with up to three other people. Beyond that, use a facilitator.

Starting the session: dedicated space: I like to begin this process by creating a sense of focus and safety in the space that I or we are using. The ways I do this include:

- Visualising a sphere of golden light around the space we're using and the people in it.
- Lighting a candle, and stating my aim for the session as I do so, hence the candle embodies my intention.
- Praying for guidance and support. For example, if I'm trying to make sense of a conflict in a project team, I'd call

for support from the Angel of Reconciliation, the Angel of Understanding, and from the spirit or guiding essence of the project itself.

Recording: you need some way to capture what's said in the session, as you'll never remember all the detail. Ideally, make an audio recording, and go through it later to write up any notes. Or if you have someone supporting you, ask them to take notes during the session, and pause periodically to help them keep up.

Starting the session: stating your intention: I find it makes quite a difference to state your aim for the session out loud, at least once. The way I'd explain this is that it helps to call in subtler sources of insight, so my intuition can identify less obvious voices which need to be heard.

Picturing the circle: this is where the session really begins. I'd advocate visualising a circle of seats, around a campfire or round table. What's important is to create an atmosphere that is inclusive and equal, so picture your circle as a place where all voices are welcome, including surprise visitors, and where there is no hierarchy. See yourself as the host who hears all speakers with equal respect.

Inviting the voices: you could start by naming the voices in the situation which you're already aware of. It's good to do this aloud, and then follow your intuition about the order they speak in. For example, if this is a conflict in a project team, there may be one or two people you feel at odds with. You might also name voices for a couple of aspects of the project itself, such as its vision or ideals, the operational reality, the finances, the clients.

You may want to name two or three voices to express aspects of yourself: for example, what you ought to do, what your fun-loving side would do, what your hurt feelings are saying. And you could call on voices for higher guidance, such as an Angel quality, or a spiritual guide like Jesus, Buddha or Mother Meera.

Speaking from the voices: when you're ready to start talking as a particular voice, pause before you start. Take a few deep breaths, and try to empty your mind of thoughts. Close your eyes, and give yourself over to this voice. Let your body posture, and body language, align with it. Imagine you *are* this voice, let it take you over, notice what its emotions are, let your face express them. You may have to wait a little, but let words flow through you, don't just try to imagine them. When you've finished speaking as that voice, it may help to stand up, shake your body, and say out loud, 'I release my identification with the voice of. . .' And thank this voice for its help.

Surprise guests: at any stage in the process, and certainly after you've gone through your initial list of voices, pause and observe if there are any other voices which need to be heard. These may be the ones that are shy, angry, doubtful that you want to hear them. Accept that they may need coaxing or reassuring to be willing to speak, and their views might not be gracefully put or easy to hear. Thank them anyway.

Confusion and synthesis: The Circle of Voices has parallels with the Diamond Process in Chapter 4. Don't worry if partway through, you feel overwhelmed and confused by lots of voices which seem to contradict each other. When you believe all the voices have been heard, give space for a synthesis, a resolving insight, to emerge. Have a silent pause, a tea break, or a short walk, and stay open to intuitive responses bubbling up. You might need to go back and check with some voices to help you reach a robust conclusion.

Completion: it's important to wrap up a session like this a bit formally, just as you began it. Give thanks to all the voices who have spoken, release any qualities, Angels, guiding spirits that you called in at the start. Dissolve the protective sphere of light. Blow the candle out as part of your completion.

Facing the 2020s: Community Insights

This is a short overview of a research project which I initiated in 2011–13 on UK community resilience, which still offers some useful insights.

The research was led by Reos Partners, a non-profit consultancy who specialise in enabling innovation in complex social systems, working with a wide range of stakeholders, including private, public sector and community organisations. Their work included over 30 diagnostic interviews, extensive desk research, and exploratory workshops in London, Edinburgh and Cardiff with potential stakeholders, including national and local government, NGOs and community organisations.

Key Insights

1. *Reproductivity:* On most aspects of community resilience, there are good exemplar projects somewhere in the UK. Why have these not been widely reproduced? One reason is that many good community resilience initiatives have depended on a few superhuman people. How can such interventions be systematised so that regular humans could implement them in a bigger number of communities? Recording what was done in an accessible toolkit form would help a lot.

2. *Sustainable funding:* Many good initiatives have also depended on funding that was not reproducible, e.g. a slab of one-off grant funding as part of a pilot programme by a charitable foundation. Sustainable funding sources could include raising capital from local communities themselves, or a social enterprise model, or even finding ways that such projects could earn a return for a private sector player.

3. *Professional services:* Often community projects struggle to find professional support geared to their particular needs, in finance, legal, property, human resources and other areas. The emergence of specialists for this sector would greatly assist reproducibility.

4. *Wider participation:* Many places don't have a strong sense of community, and in most of those that do, only a tiny percentage of people participate actively in community matters. How could larger numbers of communities, and larger numbers of people, have a motivation to participate in community resilience? Starting from basic, shared concerns is one way. Skills building and programmes like *Future Conversations* would also help.

5. *Building national resilience:* Most approaches towards community resilience take place at a geographic community level, or involve statutory organisations or charities working with local geographic communities that face particular challenges. However, examples from UK history and elsewhere show benefits in national-level approaches towards resilience. Some of the countries that are considered the most resilient, such as Japan, Norway, Sweden and Denmark, have strong national resilience policies.

6. *Working with minority groups and communities of identity:* Some communities will be more vulnerable to shocks than others, and history tells us that unresolved social tensions bubble up at times of stress. Resilient societies and communities manage to combine diversity and social cohesion. Working explicitly on community resilience creates an opportunity to pre-empt more ruptures to social cohesion that are likely to arise in economic uncertainty and rising unemployment. It is important to involve minority communities in the resilience journey, and communities of identity such as LGBT, instead of focussing solely on geographic communities.

7. *Online resilience services:* Particularly useful would be a website through which people could quickly and safely

connect with others around a given social or environmental issue in their area. For example, if you wanted to find out more about local energy initiatives, you could search all of the initiatives being developed across the UK and contact those involved, plus find contacts near you. Such tools and information could empower communities to find locally owned solutions.

8. *Engaging local authorities:* As funding for services has moved from central government to local authorities, many local authorities have sought to devolve decision-making and budgetary decisions to local communities. This means that in some parts of the country, local communities are strongly engaged with the local authority, and structures exist to support these partnerships. This move towards greater local control highlights the potential to tackle many priorities (environmental, public service reform, etc.) by adopting a resilience approach and involving local people in community action and resilience building. In recent years, some local authorities have become real innovators in new forms of service delivery, partnership working and more. Most local authorities are desperately short of funds to meet the demands on them, but a partnership response with their local communities is still beneficial.

9. *Engaging the business sector:* Large institutions and the private sector tend to be absent from discussions on improving resilience. However, shocks have a huge impact on businesses; for example, the high number of insurance claims following floods. Important opportunities can be found in exploring the role of business in developing resilience among individuals and communities, including new technologies and services.

Acknowledgements

The roots of this book grow from the two Nature-based charities I founded back in the 1990s: Magdalen Farm and Hazel Hill Wood. Both projects have involved dozens of devoted staff over the years, and both have helped thousands of visitors.

At Magdalen Farm I especially thank my co-founding trustees, Giles Chitty and Janice Dolley, and the farming teams who got us started and taught me so much: Richard van Bentum and Lya Koornneef, and Peter Foster and Christina Ballinger.

At Hazel Hill Wood, Agatha Rodgers had a crucial role in my spiritual connection, and Robin Walter and Jason Turner taught me about sustainable forestry and conservation. In recent years, Marcos Frangos, Maddy Harland, Jake Farr and Oliver Broadbent have all helped to fulfil our vision of wellbeing and resilience through Nature connection.

The third place which has inspired this book is our garden at home. I am hugely grateful to my wife Linda for the love, intelligence and hard work she brings to our garden, and for her willingness to use the methods in this book. What I brought owes a lot to the gardens at Findhorn Foundation, and to Machaelle Small Wright's Perelandra Garden.

In producing this book, my PA Carol Nourse has been invaluable, and I've been supported by several close friends as birth companions: Nayyer Hussain, Marcos Frangos and Jane Sanders, plus encouragement from many friends and wider contacts. I also want to appreciate Francis Blake and Martha Heppell-Joyce for checking my organic references, and my wife Linda and daughters Ella and Frances for all their love and support. The fruit of this book has a long history, and I hope it ripens further with you, the reader.

About Alan Heeks

Alan Heeks is an inspiring guide to helping people cultivate their wellbeing through parallels with Nature. After a Harvard MBA and successful career managing building materials businesses, Alan has spent 30 years creating Nature-based learning venues, and leading groups there.

In 1990, he started Magdalen Environmental Trust, converting 130 acres to a mixed organic farm and education centre. Since 1992 he has created Hazel Hill Wood as a 70-acre conservation wood and retreat centre. Alan has led many workshops with his Seven Seeds of Natural Happiness approach, for individuals, community groups and NHS doctors. Since 2017, Alan's workshops and writing have focussed on resilience and climate change. His non-profit organisation, Seeding our Future, has initiated a number of innovative pilot projects, including climate adaptation and food security for communities, and Nature Resilience Immersions for hospital doctors and GPs.

Alan's climate response work includes not only local community projects in the UK, but also ongoing involvement with the Deep Adaptation Forum, and support for initiatives in East Africa, where he has worked as a volunteer with the charity Farm Africa.

Personal and spiritual development groups have helped Alan's growth, and have been a focus for many groups he has led. This includes ten retreats in the Tunisian Sahara, travelling by foot and camel with Bedouin guides. He has also co-led several men's groups and creative ageing workshops, leading to his books on these themes.

Alan's leisure interests include music of many kinds, steam railways, literature, walking and cycling. He and his wife Linda are keen gardeners, and grow much of their food in their garden at home.

Keep Growing with Alan

If you've enjoyed this book, here are some ways you can get further insights, event news and updates from Alan.

Natural Happiness newsletter: this free e-newsletter comes out every couple of months, including new blogs, events, book reviews and more. To receive it go to **www.naturalhappiness. net/newsletters**

Websites: these sites provide information on different areas of Alan's activities:

www.naturalhappiness.net: this covers some of the approaches in the book, plus a lot of additional resources, including short videos. You can contact Alan via this website.

www.seedingourfuture.org.uk: updates on a range of projects and resources to help communities, individuals and NHS health professionals with resilience to climate change and other ongoing challenges. Plus resources on community-building.

www.alanheeks.com: mainly about Alan's books and articles, especially those on creative ageing, plus blogs about trains, football, and lots more besides.

www.soulresilience.net: this offers insights, processes and blogs to help you raise your spiritual resilience and find a bigger perspective on life's perplexities.

www.living-organically.com: think of this website like a rarely visited hermit's cabin in a remote, scenic valley. It offers wisdom insights from Alan's Sahara retreats, from Sufi teachers, forests, and various other sources.

Other Books by Alan Heeks

Not Fade Away: Staying Happy When You're Over 64

The late sixties and beyond are a landmark: a good time to choose what you want from the years ahead, and take stock of the story so far. This short, practical book offers you the new skills, information and resources to help you to be happy in your vintage years.

The book has three sections: *Finding your Gifts* helps you recognise and value where you are now, and gain new skills like inspiration and reinventing friendship. *Digging the Challenges* offers positive, practical ways to face into issues like health and money. *Fresh Maps* brings different ways to see life at this age as an adventure, with wisdom from various sources.

You can buy *Not Fade Away* as a paperback or ebook via Amazon and other online channels, or from Alan direct.

Out of the Woods: A Guide to Life for Men Beyond 50

Midlife and beyond can be the most fun a man has ever had, but it's also a time for fresh skills and a new path. When the roles that define men dissolve — work, marriage, fatherhood — it's a time of huge possibility and freedom, but it's easy to feel lost in the woods, with nowhere to turn to.

This book is a guide for men beyond 50: complete with route-finder, service areas, scenic highlights and emergency callout advice. It gathers the best wisdom and experience of many men on the skills you need to handle the losses and shipwrecks, and find your way out of the woods. This book has also proved helpful for many women beyond 50, both in exploring their own midlife, and understanding the men around them.

This friendly book offers insights, inspiration, practical advice and resources for further help. The basic aim is simple: enjoy your best years to the full! *Out of the Woods* provides guidance you might expect, and some to surprise you. Alan shares his experience and others' about renewing relationships, job changes, ageing parents and lots more, plus there's a chapter on health issues by a holistic doctor. But this book also offers wisdom from the unexpected, like a Wiltshire wood, Sufi mystics, football, car maintenance, and heroic myth.

Available as a paperback from bookshops, online channels or from Alan direct.

The Natural Advantage: Renewing Yourself

This pioneering book translates the principles and practices of organic farming to show how individuals, teams and organisations can grow their resilience to stress, change and uncertainty, and improve their effectiveness and wellbeing at work. *The Natural Advantage* uses largely the same basic model as *Natural Happiness*, but focussed on organic farming and the workplace, not organic gardening and personal and community wellbeing.

Alan comments, 'There has been huge progress in understanding environmental sustainability in recent decades, but few people recognise that there are similar issues around human sustainability. The human resources in many work organisations are being depleted and polluted in the drive for output: organic farming offers us a simple, vivid, practical model to change this.'

The Natural Advantage has been published in the UK, US, Netherlands, Japan and elsewhere. The UK edition: ISBN 18578826-1-X: now out of print in the UK, but available second hand.

The Find Your Gift in Work Workbook

This is an 80-page, spiral-bound A4 workbook which will guide you through a process of exploration to identify the kind of work that would really fulfil you, and make it happen. This is a self-help book with a sequence of clear processes and checklists for you to follow, helping you to value all your talents, see what you really want, test drive your fantasy, and find the right opportunities.

Available by mail from Alan Heeks: for price and contact form, see **www.alanheeks.com**

O-BOOKS

SPIRITUALITY
O is a symbol of the world, of oneness and unity; this eye represents knowledge and insight. We publish titles on general spirituality and living a spiritual life. We aim to inform and help you on your own journey in this life.
If you have enjoyed this book, why not tell other readers by posting a review on your preferred book site?

Recent bestsellers from O-Books are:

Heart of Tantric Sex
Diana Richardson
Revealing Eastern secrets of deep love and intimacy to Western couples.
Paperback: 978-1-90381-637-0 ebook: 978-1-84694-637-0

Crystal Prescriptions
The A-Z guide to over 1,200 symptoms and their healing crystals
Judy Hall
The first in the popular series of eight books, this handy little guide is packed as tight as a pill bottle with crystal remedies for ailments.
Paperback: 978-1-90504-740-6 ebook: 978-1-84694-629-5

Shine On
David Ditchfield and J S Jones
What if the aftereffects of a near-death experience were undeniable? What if a person could suddenly produce high-quality paintings of the afterlife, or if they acquired the ability to compose classical symphonies? Meet: David Ditchfield.
Paperback: 978-1-78904-365-5 ebook: 978-1-78904-366-2

The Way of Reiki
The Inner Teachings of Mikao Usui Frans Stiene
The roadmap for deepening your understanding of the system of Reiki and rediscovering your True Self.
Paperback: 978-1-78535-665-0 ebook: 978-1-78535-744-2

You Are Not Your Thoughts.
Frances Trussell
The journey to a mindful way of being, for those who want to truly know the power of mindfulness.
Paperback: 978-1-78535-816-6 ebook: 978-1-78535-817-3

The Mysteries of the Twelfth Astrological House
Fallen Angels
Carmen Turner-Schott, MSW, LISW
Everyone wants to know more about the most misunderstood house in astrology — the twelfth astrological house.
Paperback: 978-1-78099-343-0 ebook: 978-1-78099-344-7

WhatsApps from Heaven
Louise Hamlin
An account of a bereavement and the extraordinary signs —
including WhatsApps — that a retired law lecturer received from
her deceased husband.
Paperback: 978-1-78904-947-3 ebook: 978-1-78904-948-0

The Holistic Guide to Your Health & Wellbeing Today
Oliver Rolfe
A holistic guide to improving your complete health, both inside
and out.
Paperback: 978-1-78535-392-5 ebook: 978-1-78535-393-2

Cool Sex
Diana Richardson and Wendy Doeleman
For deeply satisfying sex, the real secret is to reduce the heat, to
cool down. Discover the empowerment and fulfilment of sex with
loving mindfulness.
Paperback: 978-1-78904-351-8 ebook: 978-1-78904-352-5

Creating Real Happiness A to Z
Stephani Grace
Creating Real Happiness A to Z will help you understand the
truth that you are not your ego (conditioned self).
Paperback: 978-1-78904-951-0 ebook: 978-1-78904-952-7

A Colourful Dose of Optimism
Jules Standish
It's time for us to look on the bright side, by boosting our mood
and lifting our spirit, both in our interiors, as well as in our closet.
Paperback: 978-1-78904-927-5 ebook: 978-1-78904-928-2

Readers of ebooks can buy or view any of these bestsellers by
clicking on the live link in the title. Most titles are published in
paperback and as an ebook. Paperbacks are available in
traditional bookshops. Both print and ebook formats are available
online.

Find more titles and sign up to our readers' newsletter at
www.o-books.com

Follow O books on Facebook at **O-books**

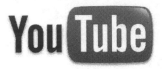

For video content, author interviews and more, please subscribe to our YouTube channel:

O-BOOKS Presents

Follow us on social media for book news, promotions and more:

Facebook: O-Books

Instagram: @o_books_mbs

Twitter: @obooks

Tik Tok: @ObooksMBS